Dyslexia Over the Lifespan

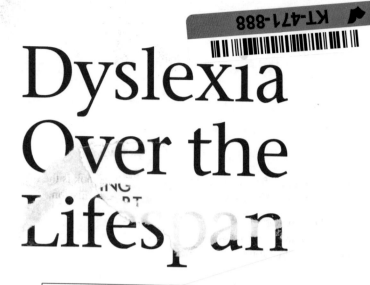

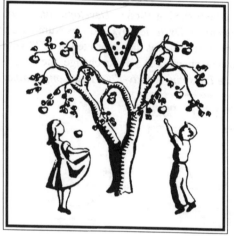

A FIFTY-FIVE-YEAR LONGITUDINAL STUDY

Margaret B. Rawson

Educators Publishing Service, Inc.
Cambridge, Massachusetts

The drawing that first appears on the cover of this book is the official logo of
The School in Rose Valley, and is reprinted with permission.

The School in Rose Valley
20 School Lane
Rose Valley, PA 19063

This book was first published in 1968 as *Developmental Language Disability:
Adult Accomplishments of Dyslexic Boys* and was Number 2 in the Hood
College Monograph Series. It was then reprinted in 1978 with a new preface.
In 1995, with four new chapters and a title change, the book is being published
as *Dyslexia over the Lifespan: A Fifty-Five-Year Longitudinal Study.*

Educators Publishing Service, Inc.
31 Smith Place
Cambridge, MA 02138-1000

Library of Congress catalog number 95-60581

ISBN 0-8388-1670-3

To
Peter Scott Olmsted
1924–1962

The source and inspiration of this study, but for whose valiant struggles with the problems of Specific Language Disability the work here presented would not have come about.

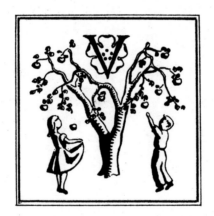

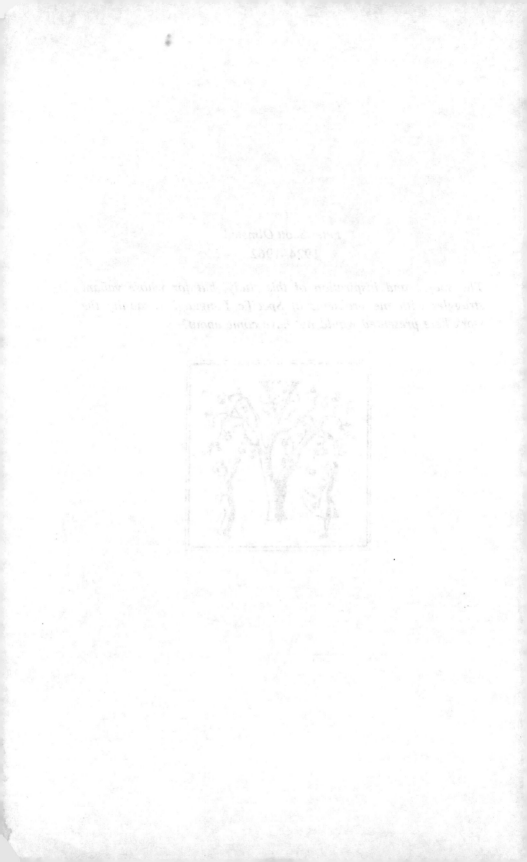

ACKNOWLEDGMENTS

The desirability of making informally gathered information into a more extended, formal study of the educational and vocational careers of this group of boys was first suggested by Professor Ralph C. Preston, Associate Dean, Graduate School of Education, University of Pennsylvania. The formulation of the plan of comparison of the dyslexic with the non-dyslexic boys as here undertaken was made under the guidance of Dr. Richard L. Masland, Director of the National Institute of Neurological Diseases and Blindness, and the study was carried out with his continued encouragement and advice.

The work was partially supported by a grant from the National Easter Seal Research Foundation. Without their help the project could not have been carried out. To Hood College, for giving the volume its financial support and its acceptance for publication in its Monograph Series—this is officially Volume No. 2, Hood College Monograph Series—the author is especially indebted.

Miss Grace Rotzel, Principal of The School in Rose Valley since its beginning, stood behind the writer's efforts to help the boys while in school and more recently has given enthusiastic support to this study. The members of the staff of the school in 1964–1965 were most helpful and encouraging. The interested participation of the boys themselves, now young men, and of their wives, parents, brothers, sisters and others who knew them, from New England to California, made the gathering of the data not only possible but a highly pleasurable experience. To all of these people I express my warmest appreciation.

Looking further back in time, the debt of the author, the school, and the boys to the late Dr. Samuel T. Orton, Dr. Paul Dozier, and Miss Anna Gillingham; and to Mrs. June L. Orton of the Orton Reading Center, Mr. Gillet Ketchum of the Re-education Clinic, Pennsylvania Hospital, and to many others will be apparent to the readers, a debt gratefully acknowledged by the author.

Dr. John Money of The Johns Hopkins University School of Medicine has been a helpful critic; the warmth of his encouragement and his generosity of time and attention to the improvement of the manuscript are especially appreciated.

The friends who have acted as editorial assistants, especially Dr. E. Carleton MacDowell, Jane W. Wise, and Phebe W. Summers have rendered not only the writer but the readers great service in improving the accuracy and clarity of the work. Mary W. Masland's helpful criticism and warm support and encouragement are particularly appreciated. Mary S. Elkins has borne tolerantly, cheerfully, and efficiently with the vicissitudes of manuscript preparation. Other colleagues have helped in many ways, especially with preparation of figures and with guidance in statistical analysis.

Parts of the material have already appeared in the *Academic Therapy Quarterly* and the *Bulletin of The Orton Society*. Their permission for reprinting and the permission of Harcourt, Brace and World, Inc. and of the Parents Bulletin of The School in Rose Valley for use of quotations are acknowledged with thanks. Thanks are also due to the school and to the artist, Eleanor P. Mather, for permission to use the school emblem.

Errors, faults of judgment, and sins of omission rest, of course, on the shoulders of the author.

Margaret B. Rawson

Frederick, Maryland
1967

1995 ACKNOWLEDGMENTS

From beginning to end, this book has been supported most substantially by generous gifts of time and effort supplied by many friendly people who have thus shown both personal kindness and belief in the project's worth. I have been exceptionally fortunate in this respect. Additionally, a financial grant from the Anna Gillingham funds of the Orton Dyslexia Society was not only an aid in the preparation of the manuscript, but also a most welcome vote of confidence.

I would like to thank the people whose interest and involvement have continued from the earlier part of the study: the men who are its subjects and who responded so cooperatively to my inquiries, as did their families and friends in The School in Rose Valley community. The men's generosity in time and good will have made what might have seemed excessive requests or intrusiveness into occasions of friendly renewal. My warm thanks are extended also to several teachers and others at the school whom I have known over the more recent years, notably Edith Klausner, the school's principal in the 1980's, and Ruth Goodenough, who was responsible for the school's 1986 alumni survey.

People in my wider fields have made possible and actual the concluding chapters of this study, continuing the story begun so many years ago. I feel that I have been part of a large group of friends who are experts and experts who are friends, and I am most grateful to them. Each is remembered and sincerely appreciated, although space permits mention by name of only a few who must represent them all. Consultation with supportive colleagues has been helpful to me as an independently operating researcher. I have need of their interest, encouragement, and, from time to time, their critical review or reappraisals from their different areas of expertise.

Special thanks are due to Dr. Richard Masland who has continued to review this manuscript and make helpful suggestions. It has also been my privilege to know personally other scientists to whose work I have referred in the book. They have deepened by understanding, and I am mindful of how much I owe them. People have given me help in innumerable ways that I will not try to categorize, but here I do want to express appreciation by name particularly to: Roger Saunders, John Bigelow, Norman Geschwind, Paula Rome, William Ellis, Rosa Hagin, Carl and Carol Kline, Edith LaFrance, Alice Koontz, Roger Shaw, Betty Levinson,

Claire Nissenbaum, Joyce Steeves, Marcia Henry, Diana King, Priscilla Vail, Valerie Beatts, Marcia Mann, Stephen Wilkins, Jan Paul Miller, and Martin Chamberlain. In this book, as elsewhere, Sylvia Richardson has been at my elbow whenever I have needed her wise counsel or editorial help and fine-tuning, right to the end of the preparation of this text for publication. There is simply no way in which adequately to express my enduring gratitude to my warm friend and quite irreplaceable multi-skilled associate, Charlotte Chamberlain. We have worked long and well together. Each of these people knows the special ways in which he or she has contributed to my work in timely, often crucial, fashion. To them, individually and collectively, my debt is enormous.

Above all, I give thanks to my loving family. That they have borne cheerfully and patiently with my long absorption in this project is but one of the ways in which they enrich my life.

My publishers, Robert and John Hall of Educators Publishing Service, have been perennially encouraging and friendly in their acceptance of my foibles and delays. I very much appreciate the skill with which they have expedited seeing this volume into print.

Margaret B. Rawson

Frederick, Maryland
February 1995

CONTENTS

FIGURES

TABLES

PROLOGUE

AN OVERVIEW FROM 1990

Dyslexia over the Lifespan: A Fifty-Five-Year Longitudinal Study is a revised and enlarged edition of *Developmental Language Disability: Adult Accomplishments of Dyslexic Boys*, published in 1968[1] by The Johns Hopkins Press (Rawson, 1968), reprinted in 1978, and kept in print by this edition's publisher, Educators Publishing Service, Inc.

This prologue to the book has two initial messages for its readers. One of these is to give a brief overview of the whole story so that the reader has a basic framework in which to consider it. The second point is to indicate how and why both the content of the story and the mode of the presentation are designed to encourage the reader to resist the temptation of reading the new material in the later chapters first.

As we introduce this book's second edition, with its additional concluding chapters, a brief summary may be in order, calling attention to some particulars of the study's development and the theory and practice that accompanied them.

The whole account, as the title indicates, covers a time span of fifty-five years in a period of accelerating cultural change. The pattern of the book reflects the complexity of its subject matter as it weaves together the strands of its subjects' lives against their changing backgrounds. The study focuses on 56 boys who attended The School in Rose Valley in the 1930's and 1940's, and the men they later became.

In this second edition of the book the first six chapters have been reprinted verbatim from the 1968 volume (Rawson, 1968). These are followed by new chapters covering intervening events, especially as brought

---

[1] The account that was published in 1968 was based on a study that was conducted by the author in 1965. Both dates are referenced in the text.

to light by the 1990 follow-up findings. The best way to understand the entire story is to read the reprinted chapters of Part I first, even if this requires rereading by one already familiar with the original study. That reading seems to call for a quick, stage-setting overview of what lies behind the more detailed account and analysis that make up the 1935 to 1990 segment of human history recounted in the ensuing chapters.

The opening scene is set in Moylan, Pennsylvania, at The School in Rose Valley, an independent, elementary school for boys and girls[2] which celebrated its 60th anniversary in 1989. From the beginning, it was part of the Progressive Education Movement and was established by a self-initiated group of parents with the guidance of the Department of Education of nearby Swarthmore College. The school was, and still is, managed and maintained by parents and staffed by professional educators assisted by qualified parents. The parent community, high in talent and commitment but low in funds, enriched the curriculum with special teaching and doubled financial resources with cooperative labor. The financial stringencies of the Great Depression and World War II taxed adult ingenuity and determination, leaving no room for luxury. The school has always presented a varied, rich, holistic, structured curriculum and ethos, rather than an excessively permissive atmosphere. It is committed to meeting the individual and social needs of its children. An excellent account of its history, philosophy, and practice was engagingly written by Grace Rotzel who was principal of the school for its first thirty-seven years (Rotzel, 1971).

In 1935, within this framework, the school and I were introduced to the work of Samuel T. Orton, M.D., then a practicing neuropsychiatrist in New York City, to help us meet the special requirements of a particular nonreading student. He diagnosed the boy as having a "specific developmental language disability," now called dyslexia. The prescribed treatment was so successful that it came to be used for the remediation of reading and other language difficulties throughout the school, at first under the guidance of Dr. and Mrs. Orton and especially of their associate, Dr. Paul Dozier, then practicing at the Pennsylvania Hospital in Philadelphia. The recommended procedures closely followed those devised by Samuel Orton, Anna Gillingham, a psychologist, and Bessie Stillman, a master teacher. Still tailored to individual needs, this is substantially what

[2] See pp. 13–14 for the explanation of why girls are not included in this study.

is today known as the "Orton/Gillingham Approach." Much of its theoretical basis is discussed in the original 1968 text which is here reprinted.

As a teaching staff member at The School in Rose Valley, I carried out and developed the program, with its accompanying testing and case-finding, until 1947 when I left. This language development program was then well ahead of its time, both theoretically and pragmatically. During this period I was developing a personal career in research and practice in the language acquisition field, and I was keeping records of student work and measured progress for future reference. Years later these notes provided invaluable aids to the accuracy of this volume.

Our analysis continues to be one of a small number of extensive longitudinal studies of the learning process and its outcomes, with special references to reading and the related skills and functions of language. It is, and perhaps always will be, unique because the circumstances which made its experimental design possible are unlikely to be repeatable, either by chance or by intent. Not only has the time span been exceptionally long, but the author has been personally involved during the whole extended period that comprises the last twelve of her seventeen years at The School in Rose Valley and the forty-three succeeding years leading up to the 1990 appraisal.

The characteristics of the group which made a comparison study possible were fortuitous and unlikely to occur again. While this was an exceptional community with peculiarly appropriate conditions for investigation, the problem on which the study sheds light is a universal one; language is a large element in the distinctiveness of the human species. Much has been learned here which is applicable in other, even quite different, educational, socioeconomic, and personal settings. I have found this applicability in my own clinical and educational work with a wide variety of children, older young people, and adults. Reports from others in the field are increasingly in agreement with these findings.

In the years of this book's life it has been my privilege to observe and be active in the field, and to confer with colleagues and others in many different places around this country and abroad, and to read widely among their excellent writings. They continue to report a great deal about what is being learned and how much is still unknown. I have sifted through some of these findings so as to reduce them to writings of my own, as for example in *The Many Faces of Dyslexia* (Rawson, 1988).

At The School in Rose Valley, however pervasive as it sometimes was in the lives of individual children, the mastery of fundamental language skills was only part of the mosaic of these children's day-to-day experiences. A school as unusual as this one, combined with its then unfamiliar way of meeting language problems, intensified many adults' perennial anxieties about their children's futures.

The records, historical materials, and teachers' reports enabled a reasonably accurate ranking of each of the included students on a composite Language Learning Facility Scale devised specifically for this study. On this scale an estimate of each student's capacity for acquisition of the skills needed for language mastery was represented. The boys in the study ranged relatively continuously from those to whom language came easily—the "eulexic" ones—to those at the "dyslexic" end of the scale who had great difficulty in mastering the skills of their first language, just as Orton might have predicted.

In the 1965 analysis, a division of the whole group into three parts seemed appropriate. Twenty students in the high-aptitude and sixteen in the medium section thus provided thirty-six control subjects in two groups for comparison with the low group of twenty students who had the greatest language-learning ineptitude. On the basis of clinical examinations in childhood, the latter were categorized as moderately to severely dyslexic.

In 1965 we could use years of schooling completed as a measure of academic achievement which could be treated statistically. All of the men were secondary school graduates, and almost all of them went on to undergraduate and graduate study. Many of the men pursued master's and doctoral degrees. The resulting average for all fifty-six men was 5.7 university years completed, with some study still underway. The educational achievement graph on page 76 gives details. Informal observation had led me to expect the scores' clustering around this population mean. Surprisingly, however, the subgroup averages differed in an unexpected direction, showing 5.4, 5.7, and 6.0 years of study completed, for the high, medium, and low groups, respectively. The differences were not quite large enough to be statistically significant; that is, they could perhaps have resulted from chance factors in groups of this size. Still, contrary to conventional expectation, the dyslexics had done at least as well as their more linguistically talented schoolmates. In 1990, the final figures were 5.4, 5.7, and 6.3. Obviously the differences in the subgroup means are now even greater and help reinforce the claim that dyslexia need not be the crucial cause of academic failure.

On a standardized occupational rating scale in use in 1965, the dyslexics had a slight numerical edge in the whole group's generally favorable socioeconomic rating. Although the original rating scale is now obsolete, the occupational standings of the men have remained approximately constant as their professional lives have continued.

The study's account has much to say about the accomplishments of these men in both statistical and human terms. It tells how dyslexia and some residual problems have affected them in terms of their achievements, personal enthusiasms, satisfactions, and the general quality of their lives.

The data presented in the 1968 report claimed no more than to demonstrate, as far as one carefully examined project could do so, that *no child needs to fail because of dyslexia.* In the long run, even severely dyslexic children can be as free to pursue their life goals as their circumstances and other talents permit, and with more joy and less discomfort than is so frequently recounted. Early diagnosis and reasonably effective educational treatment are both within the capability of schools and may be critical factors in successful outcomes, as has been shown in this instance.

During their childhood, it had seemed important to understand the global and specific educational needs of our School in Rose Valley students. By adulthood some outcomes had become clear, interesting both to those who had been involved and to others who wanted to know, but the 1965 study was an unfinished serial story. Interested dyslexia-watchers can now read the new chapters to see how the story is turning out.

These men are to be seen as a singular, delimited group only in my longitudinal research stream; otherwise each belongs to his separate individual background. Here they come together in the story in three cross-sectional views: first as children in elementary school, next as younger adults in 1965, and finally as older adults around retirement age in 1990. The personal reality behind the facts and statistics is illustrated by varied case history material with paragraphs, vignettes, and cross-references taken from school records, interviews, letters, and other information gathered during my years of continued interaction and contact with the subjects themselves and with others in their milieu. Looking broadly, yet through a lens tinted by interest in their language development and the effect it had and was still having on their lives, I could once again study in some depth how they were faring and think further of how all this might be related to their early aptitude or ineptitude in mastering language.

In 1989–90, still with the subjects' enthusiastic participation, I received responses from almost all of those still living, now either retiring from their major careers or approaching the age at which they might do so. We can now see patterns in their lives that can be identified more clearly than in 1965, thanks especially to the increasing body of scientific and professional evidence in the field of dyslexia.

Personal history and scientific knowledge are particularly valuable aids in achieving insights and understanding. An unusual challenge presented here was to maintain a balance between the objectivity proper to scientific research and the continuous personal involvement without which the course I have described could not have been run. This project had its roots in that part of the children's education which was concerned with their learning of language skills. Only in the report of their adult accomplishments in 1965 did it become a research design with the author reporting as participant-observer. In a culture full of polarized dimensions in language and behavioral traits, it has been my lifelong predilection to try to understand the paradox of living with the interplay of constancy and variation. In this study, as a reasonably well-disciplined scientist and a long-time working participant in the world of the helping professions, I have tried to meld objectivity in reporting with two-way personal understanding. The significant core of this work is its focus on a specific group of very real persons by one who also has had a close eye on what has been happening within the field of dyslexia and related fields or disciplines. The study uses individual case history material, and is itself a composite case history of the group, as it interweaves this material with the theory on which it is based—as in "The Diversity Model of Dyslexia" (Rawson, 1981).

There is growing recognition of the importance of language learning differences as an aspect of the educational process. A longitudinal study such as this can shed light on language acquisition from individual, social, and personal angles, both theoretical and pragmatic in a manner as statistically scientific as can be justified by recorded observations.

As I have been able to expand my horizons and dig deeper in selected areas, realization of the soundness of the Orton-inspired foundation on which the Rose Valley experiment was based has grown progressively stronger. I speak now with what seems to me increasingly justifiable conviction about both the rationale and the pedagogical effectiveness of the approaches described in the book. I am more than grateful for the Rose Valley experience and its part in making this possible.

The late neurologist Norman Geschwind, one of my mentors, urged that we should always "keep in mind . . . the interweaving of our functional with our anatomical knowledge" (see Money, 1962). After several years of personal interchange, in 1984 just before his death, Dr.

Geschwind wrote to me in response to some questions. One of these questions was whether or not it was the redundancy in brain capacities which makes it possible for the dyslexic to function well in spite of small neural pathologies. It was his judgment as a scientist that my view of the nature of dyslexia and dyslexics was "correct in all respects." Dr. Geschwind said he believed I was the one who should say all this as "[it] is necessary *for someone who has worked directly with the dyslexic* to say it, loud and clear" (his italics). In this study's second edition I am trying to obey his mandate to say it as loudly and as clearly as I can.

The main purpose of this book, however, is summarized in the next to last paragraph of the Introduction to Part 1 (page xxiii). The realistic optimism which my findings tend to encourage has been reported by research scientists, clinicians, teachers, teachers of teachers, dyslexic students of all ages, and especially by baffled and troubled parents. It seems that the book may still be quite useful to these people. May it continue to be a factor in the promotion of personal satisfaction and the liberation of the creative potential of dyslexic learners.

INTRODUCTION

This book deals with one aspect of school failure. It focuses on the problem of inherently able boys and girls who fail to reach their potential levels of development and accomplishment because of language learning disabilities.

One aspect of this problem which clinicians and teachers face is that of prognosis. Experience of more than thirty years of work in the field of language disabilities indicates to the author that unfavorable prognoses *need not* be the correct ones, even in cases of rather severe dyslexia. Many young people she has known, starting with language learning handicaps, have become research scientists, farmers, social workers, lawyers, store managers, or whatever their other capacities permitted. This seldom happens as though by magic, or through maturation alone, or from "just faith and trying harder." The ways in which it comes about are not the primary focus of this study. The major present purpose is to report adult accomplishments in educational and occupational endeavor of one group of boys, and to do so with some degree of scientific rigor in an appraisal as free as possible from wishful thinking and unconscious selectiveness.

The author has been continuously engaged since 1935 in the examination, education, and supervision of teaching of children with specific language disabilities, now commonly called developmental dyslexia (see p. 3). These children have been attending both public and independent schools, including The School in Rose Valley, Moylan, Pennsylvania, which was the source of the present study. Experience of seven years as psychologist in a public health mental hygiene clinic, and a somewhat longer period in charge of the reading and study service for students at Hood College, Frederick, Maryland, provide the author with further breadth of background. Social casework experience at the professional level and college teaching of sociology add another dimension to her thinking. In addition to the records here examined, she has case material, including follow-up data, concerning many former students of varying ages, backgrounds, and levels of ability.

The author was identified with The School in Rose Valley in several capacities during the years from 1930 to 1947, and has maintained a close connection with it since that time. An investigator from outside the school would have been faced with fewer hazards of personal involvement, but intimate, detailed, long-term knowledge which could not have been available to such an investigator seemed to justify the risk of bias, especially since this risk was so obvious as to aid in its conscious control.

The data were derived from a population of boys attending an unspecialized school, *including both dyslexic and nondyslexic individuals* constituting an approximately continuous series with respect to language learning facility. Although this population is socially and intellectually not typical of the country as a whole, the author's other experience leads her to believe that in groups more representative of the general English-speaking population the response to adequate diagnosis and treatment might parallel that of the boys in The School in Rose Valley. The highly advantaged sector of the population which these boys represent has received less than adequate scientific attention. It is small in numbers, but its members play such important roles in our society that an intensive study of one of its typical groups seems justified.

The "clinical hypothesis" which this study first proposed to test was derived from a position commonly held among clinicians. It stated that "dyslexic students, so diagnosed between the ages of six and twelve, necessarily have substantially poorer prospects than do nondyslexic students for success in later educational and occupational achievement."

As the "statistician's null hypothesis" the same statement could be put in this way, "Given average or better intelligence, physical normality, and equivalent social and educational opportunity in both groups, differences in educational and vocational achievement by adulthood on the part of nondyslexic boys and dyslexic boys, so diagnosed between the ages of six and twelve, will not be greater than could be explained by chance alone."

There seemed to be almost no really long-term follow-up studies in this field, those of Silver and Hagin (1964), Robinson and Smith (1962), Barlow and Blomquist (1965), and Preston and Yarington (1966) being exceptions, although they were not entirely comparable, having been based on clinic populations. Perhaps the research here reported will have value as a pilot study for others dealing with representative samples or whole school populations.

If this work generates the optimism which it seems to justify (see Chapter IV), then clinicians, teachers, parents, and especially the present-day young dyslexic patients or students should feel both more hopeful and more eager to tackle the problems of specific language disability. It is for their use especially that the writer is happy to present this report.

In analysis of the data collected for the monograph, one hundred and sixteen items of information were coded onto IBM card columns, from which a large number of statistics of varying degrees of usefulness were generated; they tempted the researcher to mine for unsuspected relationships. However, because of time and budget limitations the final statistical analysis by computer was confined to sixteen of the categories which seemed most promising from initial findings; to these were added a few pencil and slide rule calculations. Unexplored territory still beckons from all directions.

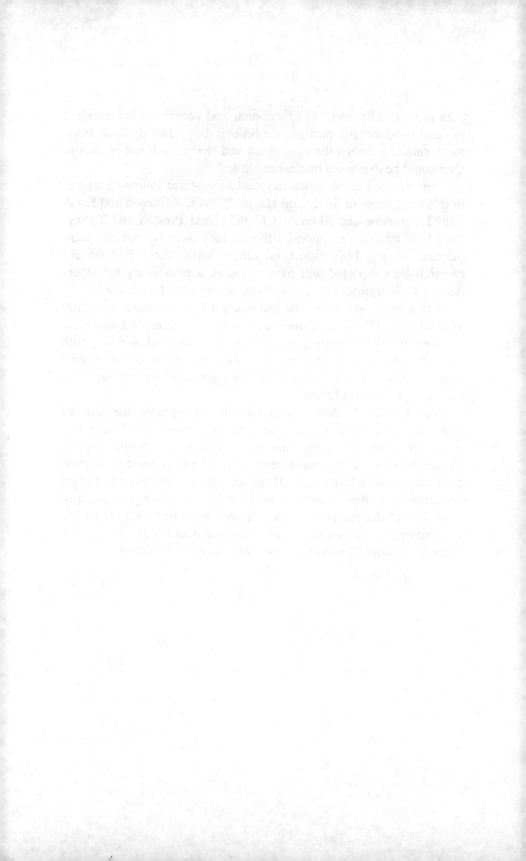

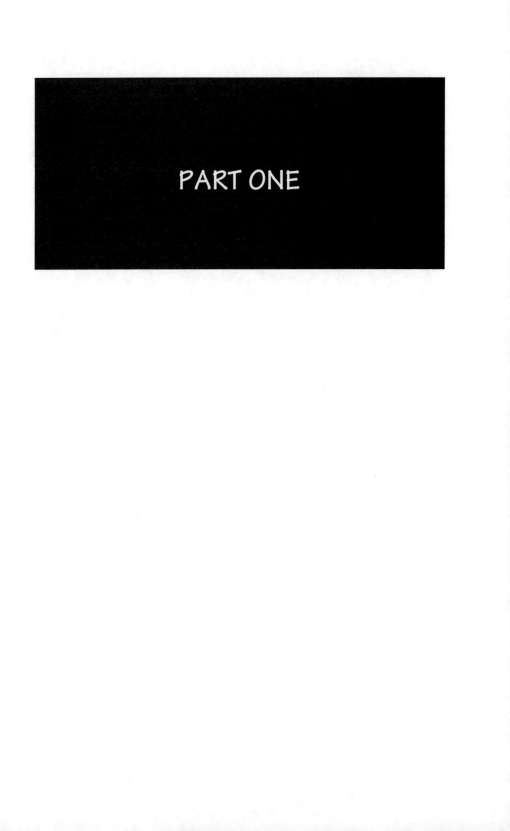

PART ONE

Chapter I

LANGUAGE—
FUNCTION AND DYSFUNCTION

The central concept of specific language disability, or dyslexia, emerges from a confluence of concerns of neurologists, psychologists, and educators. Neurologists and other physicians first noted the symptomatic similarity between aphasias resulting from injury or disease and a marked developmental delay or inadequacy in language on the part of otherwise normal individuals. This apparently constitutional disability became most evident in school failures. Psychologists and educators were first concerned with bright school children who were unable to learn to read, and with the emotional and social problems associated with this failure. As members of the various professions have pressed their search for a more complete description of the problem, knowledge of its causes, and prescriptions for its treatment, they have found themselves developing both greater breadth and more understandings in common.

The term "dyslexia" is used here in its extended meaning, as synonymous with "specific developmental *language* disability," called "strephosymbolia" (twisted symbols) by S. T. Orton because of the prevalence of orientation and sequence confusions among the persons we now call "dyslexic."[1]

Whatever the terms used, the basic definition of *developmental*

---

[1] Webster, in the Second Edition unabridged dictionary (Merriam-Webster, 1934), supports this usage: "*dys*—faulty, impaired . . . *lexis*—speech, from *legein,* Gr., to speak, confused with Lat., *legere,* to read [the medically more common interpretation, as in *alexia*] . . . *lexic,* of or pertaining to, or connected with words, or the vocabulary of a language, as distinguished from its grammar and construction." Or, as a ten-year-old rendered it with Anglo-Saxon simplicity, "What's *wrong* is my *words.* I forget them!"

3

dyslexia, as understood at the time of the diagnostic study of the boys here considered, has grown logically into that held by many present-day workers in this field. A child may be considered dyslexic within this definition if his achievement in spoken language, reading, spelling, penmanship, and perhaps other associated language skills, singly or in combination, falls appreciably below expectations based on his age, physical condition, intellectual ability (individual IQ test) and conventional educational opportunity. This is approximately the definition used not only by S. T. Orton (1925, 1928, 1937) but more recently by Hermann (1959), Gallagher (1960), Eisenberg, Money, Rabinovitch, and Saunders, in Money (1962), Critchley (1964), Cole and Walker (1964), Flower, Goffman, and Lawson (1965), J. L. Orton in Money (1966), and Thompson (1966); a collection of S. T. Orton's papers will be found in J. L. Orton (1966b).

An overall appraisal of each student seems more relevant than reliance on quantitative criterion scores alone. Deficiencies in the several language areas are seldom equal, nor, in fact, necessarily all present, in an individual. A somewhat detailed, although not exhaustive, discussion of symptoms will be found in Chapter III.

John Money (1962, p. 16) says, "It is not at all rare in psychological medicine that a disease should have no unique identifying sign, that uniqueness being in the pattern of signs that appear in contiguity. Out of context, each sign might also be encountered in other diseases, or, in different intensities, in the healthy [as in many of our own nondyslexic cases, to be described]. Specific dyslexia is no exception in this respect."

DYSLEXIA—HISTORY OF THE CONCEPT

The history of the recognition of developmental dyslexia as a constitutional problem, rather than one based in organic pathology, goes back to the work of W. Pringle Morgan in 1896 and James Kerr in that year and the year following. James Hinshelwood, who worked during the next two decades on problems of adult aphasia and on symptomatically similar childhood disabilities, published a monograph, *Congenital Word-blindness,* in 1917. While this is a careful description of symptoms, he was concerned, as are many workers today, primarily with extreme cases. He thought their problems were probably organic in nature, since they were similar in appearance to those of persons with evidence of acquired brain disease. A few other investigators, mostly English ophthalmologists as was Hinshelwood, began during this period to mention apparent hereditary factors and the prevalence of boys over girls among those affected with the condition.

In the United States it was again the ophthalmologists who at first contributed most to the recognition of the nature of developmental language disabilities. Their observations led eventually to the recognition that the difficulty lay not in the eyes but in the functioning of the language areas of the brain. From one ophthalmologist, Herman K. Goldberg, we have the statement, "Not the eye but the brain learns to read." [See Hermann (1959), p. 33.]

Psychologists and educators in the first quarter of this century with the notable exceptions of Bronner (1917) and Hollingworth (1918, 1925), extensively quoted in Thompson (1966), gave little attention to the special disabilities in the language field which had been observed by members of the medical profession. They concentrated, rather, on the reading process as seen from a pedagogical viewpoint. Parallel but generally noninteracting lines of development of medical and nonmedical interests continued, with frequent and sometimes scathing rejection of the neurological viewpoint by some psychiatrists and educators [e.g., Gates (1949)], while some clinicians failed to understand the classroom situation in the public schools. Such situations still frequently exist.

In 1925 there began in Iowa an investigation into the causes of referral of children to the mental health facilities of one of the first mobile outpatient psychiatric clinics—one which, with its "team" of psychiatrist, psychologist and social worker, sounds very modern. Dr. Samuel T. Orton, the psychiatrist of this clinic, had the added breadth of view which derived from an already long experience as a neuroanatomist and neuropathologist who had made many clinical diagnoses and detailed postmortem studies of many human brains. He was, in addition, a hospital administrator, a university department head in psychiatry and a scholar with wide-ranging vocational and avocational interests (J. L. Orton, 1966b). With this breadth of background it is not surprising that Orton was able to propose reasonable hypotheses (which was all he claimed for them) to explain the occurrence of specific language disability in many otherwise normal children who showed no evidence of organic pathology, and to devise the beginnings of procedures for the amelioration of the difficulties they experienced.

About the cause, or causes, of dyslexia there is now more knowledge than in the period 1930–1947 when the subjects of the present study were in elementary school, but still not enough to settle controversy. The author agrees with the view that a person is not dyslexic by reason of mental subnormality, sensory defect, psychotic or neurotic disturbance, or (in the vast majority of cases) demonstrable brain damage, although these conditions sometimes coexist with dyslexia. This view holds that a neurological organization factor, often familial, appears to be involved, and that it is susceptible of amelioration with appropriate teaching.

Perhaps the most controversial of Orton's postulates is the one concerning the possibility that developmental language disability arises from the delayed development of unilateral dominance of the language areas of the cortex of one hemisphere of the brain over the other in the affected individual. This dominance has long been observed in most mature persons. The manner of the individual's achievement of hemispheric dominance—whether it is wholly innate or how and at what age it is developed—still poses many questions. What, if any, connection hemispheric dominance has with learning to read is still unknown and often the subject of conjecture and heated debate. To Orton such a connection seemed a reasonable and scientifically parsimonious explanation of observed phenomena, and one which suggested treatment approaches. Refinements of laboratory and surgical techniques and the increase of knowledge in the two decades since his death, notably work reported by Penfield and Roberts (1959), Zangwill (1960), Sperry (1964), and Masland (1967), describe this problem as more complicated than could have been fully appreciated at the time of Orton's best known publication (1937), but still leave open the question of the relationship between hemispherical dominance and developmental dyslexia. Masland (1967) describes experiments that show that ". . . when an integrative function must involve both hemispheres, it is more difficult than when it can be accomplished within a single hemisphere." He writes, "These experiments provide an explanation for lateralization of language within a single hemisphere . . . [and] . . . serve . . . to accentuate how far ahead of his time [Orton] was and how perceptive were his comments regarding cerebral dominance and dyslexia."

Studies of incidence of language disabilities are sufficiently numerous and detailed [Orton (1937), Hallgren (1950), Walker and Cole (1965), etc.] to indicate strongly that there is a familial factor to be considered. Whether this is a genetic factor cannot now be demonstrated, although it can certainly be suspected, especially from the findings of consonance with respect to language disability in monozygotic (identical) twins.

It is worth reiterating that no one symptom, and no invariant pattern of symptomatology, is universally present as the *sine qua non* of the diagnosis, despite the recognizably common character of the difficulties of the group of individuals covered by the terms "dyslexia," or "specific developmental dyslexia," or related descriptive labels. (See also Chapter III.)

It was on the basis of Orton's concepts (see p. 63), modified as time passed by increasing knowledge and experience, that the language program of The School in Rose Valley was built in the years 1935–1947,[2] and as a test of the implied hypothesis concerning prognosis that the investigation of 1964–1965 was carried out.

THE NATURE OF READING AND WRITING

Reading skill is only one part of language development but because of its central importance in academic education it was the first to receive large-scale attention in the United States. On the one hand its relation to spelling and penmanship, and on the other its dependence on established skills in recognition and production of spoken language, have become manifest. These are all aspects of decoding and encoding needed for the management of the symbolic communication of ideas. The central thought processes of verbal formulation which accompany and precede understanding and expression are often less obvious because they are internal to the thinker and less apparently connected with his overt behavior.

[2] The oldest boys entered the elementary school in 1930; the remedial-preventive language program was initiated in 1935.

Verbal Language

Verbal language (see Fig. 1) is a universal human achievement which makes possible communication of information, thought, and feeling across time and distance. It makes possible much of man's capacity for abstract thinking, long range planning, and the building and transmission of culture. The relations of "animal languages" to human language, of language to thinking, and of one's own linguistic system to his world view, as well as of verbal language to other symbolic systems, such as those of art or mathematics, are all of great interest and importance but for this study they are "background to the background."

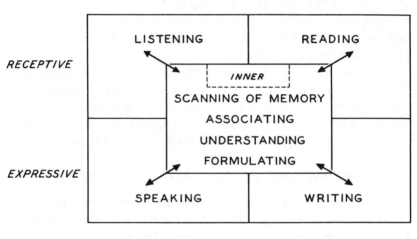

Figure 1. Verbal language. This diagram illustrates interrelationships of (a) the auditory components of language (as heard or spoken) with the visual components (as read or written); (b) the receptive aspects (listening to speech, or reading silently) with the expressive aspects (speaking and writing); and (c) the interconnection of all modalities through the cerebral activities of inner language.

Nor is this the place to consider whether the development of rational thought precedes, follows, or parallels the understanding and use of the spoken word. In the individual child's growth we often observe apparently rational behavior unaccompanied by speech and note occasions on which he obviously understands more of the speech of others than he can reproduce in his own words. Certain it is, however, that nonliterate peoples, as well as nonreading and nonwriting six-year-olds and older illiterates, normally use quite expertly in speech the linguistic systems of their mother tongues. They have learned to receive verbal messages by listening, to scan their memories for verbal form and content, to make mental associations, to understand and to be aware of such understanding, to formulate verbal messages, and to give them expression in speech. These activities are schematized very simply in Figure 1—as, respectively, "Audible, Receptive," "Inner," and "Audible, Expressive" aspects of verbal language.

Spoken (audible) language, which occurs in a time sequence, is represented in space by visible signs (in English, alphabetic-phonetic symbols in left-to-right linear sequence). This makes it possible to receive messages by reading—"Visible, Receptive" in the diagram—or to send them in writing—"Visible, Expressive." The graphic form, in English, stands for the spoken sound which, in turn, refers to event or idea, so that reading and writing are a second-order symbolization, two representational steps removed from experience.

No attempt has been made to incorporate into the diagram the sensory and motor components of language, nor to more than suggest the constant action, interaction, and integrated relationships on which language as an instrument depends. Not even a multidimensional, mobile model could do justice to the task. Sherrington (1940) might well have been describing the language processes of which he was so able a master, when he spoke of brain and mind as "an enchanted loom where millions of flashing shuttles weave a dissolving pattern, always a meaningful pattern though never an abiding one; a shifting harmony of subpatterns."

We might sum up the goal in the teaching and learning of language skills as the rapid, smooth, automatic mastery of the communicative processes for the reception and transmission of symbolic language, built on consciously acquired and retrievable systematized structure. Such mastery should lead to a sense of competence and enjoyment in linguistic activity in thought, in spoken language, and with the printed word.

Language Skills

Much of the confusion about the definition of "reading" seems to result from the two senses in which the word is commonly used. Are both parties to a discussion thinking of reading as the decoding of a printed passage into words which could be spoken (as in Figure 1, "Reading")? Or are they concentrating on the assimilation of ideas and the stimulation of thought and feeling which justify the attempt to ascertain the writer's message (part of Figure 1, "Inner Language")? Does each, in fact, know in which context the other is speaking? There could hardly be disagreement that both aspects are essential. One must decode the text accurately in order to get at the author's meaning, but word identification without under- ιtanding is at best a waste of time and at worst self-delusion.

Since we have only one word "reading" in common use, the two usages or their inclusive combination need to be specified if we are to avoid confusion in our discourse. "Does he read *easily?*" would be one way of asking, "Does he decode printed verbal symbols ac- curately and rapidly?" On the other hand, "Does he *get much out of* his reading?" might mean, "Does he understand and respond ap- propriately to the written word?" If both decoding and interpreta- tion are well-developed skills he will be likely to "read *avidly, prof- itably,* and *with enjoyment.*" "How well does he read?" is, *per se,* an ambiguous question.

Comprehension of meaning during reading varies widely from person to person, and depends on time, occasion, and subject mat- ter for any individual. Increase of understanding is a lifelong goal. The optimum use of verbal media in the service of this goal has its roots in the basic spoken language which is largely developed in the preschool years, except in circumstances of linguistic depriva- tion. Normally in the elementary school period there is added the translation of speech to and from print, with both spoken and writ- ten symbols in continuing interaction with reality as experienced by the child.

The semantic problem—the problem of meaning—was central to the whole process of education as consciously held by the school community which provided the material reported in this study. The frequent reiteration of "meaning" in connection with "reading"

would have amounted to belaboring the obvious to everyone involved, including the children. "Why else would one bother to learn
reading?" Meaning was as a matter of course considered centrally
important to reading, as to all other school experience—a generalized goal, a conscious aim.

"Writing," too, has two common meanings. Among the "three
R's" writing refers to penmanship. One needs to learn to write
freely, rapidly and legibly, if the pen is to serve the minds of both
writer and reader. But one must also have something to say and say
it effectively—the other kind of "writing"—if he wishes to convey
meaning. We can easily translate, "How well does he write?" into
either, "How good is his penmanship?" or, "Is his composition clear
and effective?"

There is also "spelling," which term is not itself ambiguous
even though it may be the least tractable of these related skills. The
right letters in the conventional order—"right writing" or "orthography"—facilitate communication by not distracting the reader's
attention from the verbal message. This is the important reason for
emphasis on spelling in the curriculum.

And so, although we write here mostly about language *skills*, the
paramount importance of *meaning* is continuously assumed as the
controlling reason for learning to use the media of expression.

DYSLEXIA AS AN EDUCATIONAL PROBLEM

It is as an impediment to the achievement of useful, enjoyable
reading and other language skills in the broad sense that specific
language difficulty or dyslexia becomes important in the child's
school life. The study of the language problems of Iowa school children previously mentioned was but the first in a long series of such
studies in which language learning difficulties have been found to be
associated with school failures and social and emotional problems,
which in turn lead to inadequate education and occupational under-
achievement.

Estimates of incidence of specific language disability among normally intelligent children who have no gross sensory defects, no major cultural deprivation or primary causative emotional disturbances,
and who have had schooling appropriate to their ages, range from

two per cent to thirty per cent, or more, of the school population; reading retardation from all causes is, of course, higher. The different estimates for the prevalence of dyslexia depend on the exact definition of the condition, the criteria used for determining adequacy (age, grade, IQ, etc.), where the estimator draws the line between adequacy and insufficiency, and how comprehensive and detailed is the testing program on which his data are based. One estimate frequently made, especially in schools serving relatively "advantaged" children, is that ten per cent will have language problems severe enough to prevent academic progress of even low-average rate, while another ten per cent will be sufficiently affected to reduce their scholastic achievement appreciably and often to convert initial enthusiasm for learning into distaste for a hard, not very rewarding, succession of tasks.

Dyslexic boys have been reported almost universally to outnumber dyslexic girls severalfold. Estimates generally given range from four-to-one to ten-to-one, and come from many countries using diverse languages. In the author's recent experience spontaneous inquiries which have come from English-speaking parents living in both Americas, Europe, Africa, and Australasia concerned thirty-nine boys but only two girls. Again, a summer reading clinic population in Claremont, California, in 1964 was composed of forty-three boys—no girls applied for admission. There are, of course, dyslexic girls; the author has known many, and their problems seem to be indistinguishable, for the most part, from those of the boys. Many conjectures, but little firm evidence, have been advanced to account for this preponderance of males, but detailed consideration of the subject is not germane to this discourse. The fact is mentioned here because it does relate to the higher incidence of dyslexia in a group of boys such as the one here studied than one would expect in a population made up of both sexes.

Chapter II

THE BOYS AND
THE SCHOOL SETTING

The subjects studied in this investigation comprise *all* of the fifty-six boys who attended The School in Rose Valley, Moylan, Pennsylvania, for at least three of their elementary school years during the period between 1930 and 1947. The total school population included other children—girls, preschoolers, and more transient attenders—but it was never large. Only fifty-six boys met the attendance criterion. *These fifty-six included nondyslexics as well as dyslexics;* being all-inclusive of their group, they can be considered a "population," rather than a "sample."

This school and period of time were chosen because the investigator was on the school staff, knew each boy and each family well, had given most of the psychometric tests and had administered and/ or analyzed all of the achievement tests which were given during the period. At least one Binet intelligence test score was available for each boy, achievement records and teachers' reports were on file, and the investigator had other records. She had made several informal follow-up studies of former students while she was still at the school and had kept in touch with many individuals. Two later follow-up questionnaire studies had been made by others at the school. It seemed likely that most of the boys could still be reached; and, in fact, contact was made with all of them in 1964–1965, either directly, through close relatives, or, in a few cases, through friends who had had very recent contact with the boys. (The primary subjects of study will always be referred to as "boys"; "fathers" are their fathers; "children," especially in Chapters IV and V, are the boys' children—the youngsters of 1964–1965.)

The school is coeducational, but this study was confined to the boys for two reasons. In the first place, here as elsewhere there were proportionately more boys than girls who were dyslexic. Since the total number was small, the dyslexic girls, while interesting on a case-study basis, would have been difficult to treat in a statistically satisfactory way. Secondly, a principal objective was to test as far as possible the limits to which the young adult subjects had been able to go in education and occupation. In our culture boys are generally more likely to approach these limits than are girls. With girls, schooling and employment outside the home take a role secondary to homemaking, and homemaking, however important, obviously cannot be graded for comparative purposes.

Should it prove possible, a study of the girls who were the contemporaries of these boys should be made. This would yield rather different data, and would round out the picture. Moreover, if there is to be further consideration of language patterns from a familial, or genetic, point of view, a follow-up study of the children of all students, both boys and girls, dyslexic and nondyslexic, would be informative.

The school has always had a nursery school and kindergarten program and forty-two of the fifty-six boys were enrolled in it for one or more years, but the study here reported had to do primarily with skills learned in the elementary grades. Three years spent in the school between first grade and sixth, or, at one period, eighth grade seemed the minimum time for validity of the investigator's judgment and for influence of the school on the boys' later careers.

To see whether the three year attendance stipulation had introduced bias into the findings, a brief examination was made of the cases of twenty-three boys who were enrolled for less than three years in the school's elementary grades and who were not, therefore, included in the study. A brief description of this group seems adequate, since they are not the main focus of attention.

Some of the twenty-three boys had been in the preschool program, others had not. All had had reading instruction; the children who had completed only first grade during the period when the school's reading instruction program began in second grade were excluded from the group of twenty-three here examined. The boys' scholastic progress during the time they were in grade school, including presence or absence of dyslexic symptoms, seemed very like that of the boys who met the attendance criterion for the study. Language problems had been identified and treated as far as time had permitted.

Reasons for the twenty-three boys' enrollment in the school seemed to be similar to those governing the choices for the fifty-six, but withdrawals were proportionately more often the result of their families' moving from the neighborhood. Among the twenty-three, six entered less than three years before their graduation. Reasons for withdrawal, other than graduation, varied, but seemed not to be disproportionately related to the boys' language status. The later histories of most of the twenty-three boys were known more or less well, although follow-up interviews with them were not part of the 1964–1965 investigation. These histories also paralleled the records of the subject population rather closely.

On all counts the boys not included seemed to be comparable to those who met the attendance criterion, so it was concluded that this limitation had probably not biased the outcome of the study.

THE SCHOOL IN ROSE VALLEY

History and Program

The School in Rose Valley, a "private" or "independent" school, was founded and operated by a pre-existing group of parents, most of whom lived within a radius of about five miles. They had been studying child development together and had developed strong agreement concerning educational objectives. The school was opened in September, 1929,[1] with three of the four oldest subjects of this study enrolled in its kindergarten class. The school operated (as it still does) on a financial "shoestring," with many scholarships and with part-time assistantships for qualified parents. Professional teachers were in charge of each grade. The period under study included the Depression and World War II. Most of the parents were professional or business people who at that time had little money. Lack of funds, however, did not appear to be a major cause of psychological strain, for all the fathers were employed and had

[1] Older readers will remember October, 1929, as the date of the financial crash which ushered in the Great Depression. Hardly the time to start a tuition-supported school!

about the same socioeconomic status. Perhaps the Depression situation in part determined the constitution of the school's very cohesive clientele. The group was not intended to be "exclusive" but circumstances produced a social homogeneity in the early years which, as it turned out, was fortunate for the purposes of the present study a generation later.

The school was designed for normal boys and girls, the high IQ range of students, again, being an accident of the constituency. It offered an inclusive curriculum in arts, natural and social sciences, crafts, and physical education. The extensiveness of the curriculum was made possible largely through the part-time work of especially qualified parents, but this did not preclude careful attention to the traditional "three R's." Ideologically, the school was part of the Progressive Education movement, attempting, as did the best of such schools, to maintain a balance of intellectual, emotional, and practical approaches to child growth and development.

The philosophy of the school community also included commitment to simultaneous attention to group life and to the nurturing of individual differences. It was as one aspect of this concern for individual differences that a program for the remediation of language difficulties was developed. The children were actively engaged in a variety of academic and nonacademic pursuits. They were accustomed to many part-time teachers of special subjects. Special attention to areas of difficulty was part of their school life, too, and felt to be only a small part even when it was intensive and regular. We are here devoting a whole book to what the children and adults knew to be only a corner of their world, however important that corner was at the time. Moreover, rapport was enhanced because the author was known to both children and teachers (and seemed to be welcome) as "academic watchdog" and consultant—who could also generally find one a good book from the library (because, as librarian, she had selected most of its volumes), or consult with a troubled parent or teacher like an unofficial school social worker (drawing on her earlier professional experience). In a sense, both children and adults were, like her, expected to be specialists at some times and generalists at others, to hold to high standards, and to the limit of their maturity self-imposed ones, on appropriate occasions. Flexibility and an experimental approach to new experience were also expected. Of course these ideals were never realized in full; but they made everyone tolerant of an individually tailored and highly structured language program, in the context of a planned but often loosely structured school life.

While there was some variation from year to year and from classroom to classroom, the basic philosophy, management, and practice of the school remained relatively constant during the years in question, so that the boys in the study shared closely similar, though of course not identical, educational experiences. Perhaps this is as close control as one can hope for, with due recognition that even small variations may be substantially important to the participants.

English Language Program

Reading instruction offered in the classrooms from 1930 through 1947 was based on the commonly used experience-chart and sight-word method, with some phonetic instruction always included. In practice the methods used in the early grades were almost identical with those now generally recommended in texts on beginning reading with basal readers, but this regime was followed as soon as possible by what would now be called "individualized reading." In the first years of the school's existence, for the 15 subjects born through 1928, reading was introduced in the first grade at about age six. Thereafter, through 1947, in the hope that an added year of maturity would speed learning and reduce failure, reading was introduced in second grade, with informal pre-reading exercises in the preceding year. The first year of reading, at whichever age, was under low pressure, with careful attention to signs of difficulty. After 1935, diagnostic testing was employed and special individual teaching was instituted when it seemed necessary, generally at the end of the first or beginning of the second year of reading instruction, that is, in late second or early third grade.

Spelling and penmanship were taught conventionally; they were often not "overlearned" by the students, even sometimes under tutoring conditions. Emphasis was on the utility of these subjects in expository or "creative" writing. Manuscript writing (printing) was taught first, with cursive script being introduced in third grade, after which each student used the form he then preferred.

Until 1935 problems in the learning of reading were met with what would now be termed "corrective reading techniques." In September, 1935, to meet the needs of our oldest subject, we were introduced to the Orton approach, described in S. T. Orton (1925, 1928, 1937) and Gillingham and Stillman (1936), and discussed more fully on pp. 63–5. This first boy was seen by Dr. and Mrs. Samuel T. Orton and Dr. Paul Dozier in New York, and a program for him and for later students was instituted at the school and continued beyond the end of the period of this study. During its first years this program was under the informal guidance of Dr. Dozier, who was then at the Institute of the Pennsylvania Hospital in nearby Philadelphia.

That there were so many children with language learning problems or needs seems explainable largely by the school's policy of attention to individual differences and by its careful screening procedures. The classroom teaching of reading, generally effective, was almost all begun with each child by the principal, then also a grade teacher, or by one very well-qualified primary teacher. Thus the variation commonly caused by staff changes was minimized (another "control" feature both fortuitous and fortunate for the present study). The probability seems to be that the staff was aware of problems which under many circumstances might not have been recognized, since it was concerned rather with individual potentials than with grade norms and was also well-informed about the various signs of language difficulty. Moreover, having been alerted to the probable familial incidence of language problems, the staff was especially alert for such patterns in siblings or cousins of known cases.

Individual instruction was given to children with varied problems other than dyslexia, and the author, in charge of the remedial program, made conscious effort not to allow enthusiasm for the Orton approach, which was so satisfactory for many children, to lead to extremes in ascribing all language learning deviance to specific language disability. In the end, the incidence of dyslexia, while high, was not out of line with the findings of the recent study of Walker and Cole (1965), where a similarly fine screen was used with a very similar population.

Careful attention to the health needs of the children largely ruled out other physical problems, and cultural deprivation did not exist. When, as occasionally happened, there were severe emotional involvements concurrent with language or more general learning problems, the specific language disability component of this complex was diagnosed as such only after suitable neuropsychiatric referral. Most of these particularly puzzling multiproblem children, and also several of the youngsters with otherwise uncomplicated language problems, were seen at the Institute of the Pennsylvania Hospital.

By and large, this school's population was representative of those of many independent schools of the Philadelphia area, though perhaps more homogeneous than most of them. In the 1935–1947 period it was one of the few schools in the United States which had a program for the diagnosis and treatment of specific language disabilities of otherwise normal children, almost a laboratory setting for investigation of school-age dyslexia, although such research was not then planned.

Most current studies concern themselves with samples representative of the general population, with the problems of groups generally or specifically disadvantaged, or with the enrichment and motivational needs of intellectually gifted children. Here was a group of intellectually gifted, culturally advantaged children from which those with language learning problems had *not* been excluded by processes of selection. This offered a probably unique opportunity: first, to study a kind of population seldom examined, but worth consideration because of its high potential; secondly, to examine the language disability children in such a group when they remained with their peers while receiving special teaching for their disabilities; and thirdly, to take advantage of a continuous acquaintance of an investigator with a group of subjects spanning a full generation's time.

FAMILY BACKGROUNDS

Homogeneity

When as few as fifty-six cases from forty-four families are to be used in two or more groups, there is considerable advantage in having a population homogeneous except for the factor under study;

fortunately this is the case here. In some ways this limits the usefulness of the results, since they cannot be representative of the region's population as a whole; but in such an inherently limited subculture group, one can study a single problem rather intensively with limited resources, generalize as far as is appropriate, and perhaps have one's work serve as a pilot study for other projects.

The forty-four families represented by the fifty-six boys of this study had much more in common than their ideas about education:

43 of the families were Caucasian; one was Oriental.

43 were Protestant or of Protestant origin; one was Jewish.

42 fathers were college graduates; one attended college without graduating; one had completed 8th grade. (There were many advanced degrees—see Table 1, and compare Table 3, Chapter III.)

43 mothers were known or presumed high school graduates; one had completed 8th grade. (There were many college and advanced degrees—see Table 1, and compare Table 3.)

43 families had both parents living and together; one father was deceased.

36 fathers were in Warner's Occupational Class I; 5 in Class II; 2 in Class III; 1 in Class IV. [See Warner (1949), pp. 140–141.]

The families were small. (Table 2)

The nontypical items were in different families, each of which was otherwise typical.

Table 1

EDUCATION OF PARENTS

44 FAMILIES OF 56 BOYS

Years Postsecondary Schooling	Fathers	Mothers
0	1	2
1 to 3	1	7
4	15	20
5	0	0
6	6	6
7	8	0
8	13	2
Unknown	0	7[a]
All parents	44	44

[a] Probably High School graduation or more.

Table 2

SIZE OF 44 FAMILIES OF 56 BOYS

Children per family	Number of families
1	9
2	20
3	12
4	2
5	1
All families	44

Parents' Involvement With the School

As has been said, the founding and operation of the school was a cooperative venture on the part of a group of parents. This cooperation continued with the physical maintenance of the plant, and with the construction of new classroom buildings by fathers, some mothers, and on one occasion by children and their shop teacher. Many mothers and occasionally a father provided special subject teaching, as well as library and other services in the interest of dollar-free curriculum enrichment or on a tuition-barter basis. The boys and girls were very much engaged in this family involvement in the school, and hence it is another facet of the close community aspect of the school's sociology and of the background of the boys in this study.

Most of the siblings of the subjects were at one time or another enrolled in the school, whether or not they figure directly in the study. Two or more, though not necessarily all, of the children in ten families are so included (see Chapter V). Thirty-three families chose the school for their children primarily because of its educational policies. This included all those having more than one son in the study. One family sought the school to meet special requirements of its older boy, enrolling the younger son because they found themselves in sympathy with the school's program; for five families it was simply "a good local private school"; for seven it answered special problem needs, in five of these cases, language learning problems. While there were some other attendance patterns, there was a strong tendency to start youngsters in the preschool and keep them enrolled, if possible, until they had reached the end of 6th, 7th or 8th grade, depending on the school's offerings at the time.

Despite their great similarity of background as just described, these fifty-six boys showed marked individual differences, as will become evident in the next chapter.

Chapter III

THE BOYS AT ELEMENTARY
SCHOOL AGE, 1930–1947

BACKGROUND

Families: Boy's-eye View

When we look at the background of the fifty-six boys in terms of their individual experiences it seems reasonable to count a "family" for each boy. Fifty-six boys experienced fifty-six fathers, mothers, and family constellations, no matter how these overlapped from the parental or census taker's viewpoints. From this point on we are interested in the forces which produced each boy, so that the basic number now shifts from the forty-four families countable by the outsider to the fifty-six backgrounds countable by the boys.

From this point of view we note of the boys that:

All were between 6 and 14 years of age when first studied at The School in Rose Valley between 1930 and 1947.

All were U.S. born, predominantly of U.S. parentage; one father was born in England; the Korean mother and father had immigrated, as the investigator recalls it, from Hawaii; the parental stock of the five adopted boys was probably also American.

55 Were Caucasian; one Oriental;

55 were of Protestant background; one was Jewish;

54 had fathers with college degrees and predominantly professional occupations (Tables 3, 4, 5).

46 had mothers who were known to have had high school or more education; 55 probably had completed high school (Tables 3, 4).

32 had mothers who worked outside the home, mostly part-time, 27 of them at the school (Table 4).

46 had fathers in Occupational Class I; 5 in Class II; 4 in Class III; one in Class IV (Table 5).

23

55 were living with both parents; one father had died; there were no divorced or separated parents.

47 boys had siblings; 9 were "only" children (Table 6).

51 boys were biological children of their parents; 5 were adopted.

Table 3

EARNED DEGREES — 56 BOYS AND THE PARENTS OF EACH BOY[a]

Degree Status	Boys[b]	Fathers[c]	Mothers[c]
Less than high school completed	0	1	1
High school graduate	0	0	1
Only noncollege schooling beyond high school	1	0	1
Graduation technical institute	1[d]	0	0
One or more years college — nongraduate	3	1	9
Studying for undergraduate degree (1964–65)	3	0	0
Teachers college diploma	0	0	1
Undergraduate degree — BA, BS, or equivalent	12	19[e]	26
Graduate study, no further degree	5	0	0
Master's or professional degree candidate	3	0	0
Master's or professional degree — MA, MS, LLB, BD, etc.	8	18	7
Study, but no degree, beyond master's level	1	1	0
Doctoral candidate	5	0	0
Doctorate — PhD, ScD, JD, etc.	8	14	3
Doctorate — Medicine	3	2	0
Postdoctoral study	2	0	0
More than one doctorate (MD and PhD)	1	0	0
Unknown	0	0	7
Total	56	56	56

[a] Parents counted once for each boy in this and all succeeding tables.
[b] As of 1964–1965.
[c] As of 1930–1947.
[d] Also attended college one year.
[e] Includes British degree in art, considered equivalent to BA.

Table 4

OCCUPATIONS — 56 BOYS AND THEIR PARENTS

Occupations	Boys	Fathers	Mothers
Doctor	2	2	0
Lawyer	4	10	0
Clergyman	0	1	0
College administrator	0	3	0
College professor	6	9	1
College instructor	1	1	0
Research scientist	8	1	0
Economist, research, consultation, or arbitration	0	4	0
Professional engineer	1	9	0
Artist, designer	0	1	0
Actor (supporting, on contract)	1	0	0
Architect	0	1	0
City planner	1	0	0
Community organization (director)	1	0	2
Social worker (in-service trained)	1	0	1
School principal	1	0	0
School teacher, MA	1	1	9
School teacher, BA	2	0	9
School teacher, no degree	1	0	8
Business, owner or manager			
Large	0	4	0
Medium	4	1	0
"Middle management" (junior executive)	7	2	0
Business, minor official	2	4	1
Sales representative, technical	3	1	0
Management trainee	1	0	0
Skilled laborer, or foreman	2	1	0
Semiskilled laborer, or apprentice	2	0	0
Housewife	0	0	25
2 or more occupations (e.g., minor business job and own medium size business)	4	0	0
Unemployed	0	0	0
Total	56	56	56

Table 5
SOCIOECONOMIC CLASS RATING — FATHERS OF 56 BOYS, 1930–1947

Socioeconomic Class	Fathers
I	46
II	5
III	4
IV	1
Total	56

Table 6
FAMILY SIZE — 56 BOYS

Children per family	Number of families
1	9
2	23
3	19
4	2
5	3
Total	56

Mean number of children — 2.4
S.D.   — 0.98

School Attendance

Of the fifteen boys born from 1924 through 1928 and the ten born from 1934 through 1938, those who completed the school's course were "graduated" at the end of sixth grade. Seventh and eighth grades were available only to those born from 1929 through 1932; after their graduation the eighth grade offering was discontinued; the boys born in 1933 were enrolled only through seventh grade.[1]

Forty-two of the boys had been in the school's nursery school and kindergarten program. Three of them were absent from Grade 1 but re-entered later.

Twelve of the boys entered after Grade 1; all of these finished

---

[1] Seventh and eighth grades were considered "elementary" at The School in Rose Valley. They were called "secondary" in schools to which the boys went next, and so appear in the follow-up data. The overlapping of categories does not influence the statistics concerned with the hypotheses being tested.

the school course. Of the other forty-four boys, four were out for a year or more but all except one, after returning, stayed to graduate. Twenty-four of the forty-four who started in first grade had six, seven, or eight of their elementary years at the school; and of the forty-two present for the first three or more years, all but three had been in the preschool program (Tables 7 and 8). Five of the twelve "late entrants" came to the school because of its language program.

On the whole, then, the boys were much more than minimally the product of the Rose Valley school experience.

Table 7

LENGTH OF ELEMENTARY SCHOOL ATTENDANCE
AT SCHOOL IN ROSE VALLEY

Number of years	Number of boys
3	8
4	11
5	9
6	19
7	3
8	6
Total	56

Mean — 5.3 years
S.D. — 1.4 years

Table 8

ELEMENTARY GRADES COMPLETED AT SCHOOL IN ROSE VALLEY

Grade completed	Beginning Grade 1	Beginning Later	Interrupted	Total
3	2	0	0	2
4	8	0	0	8
5	6	0	1	7
6	16	3	1	20
7	2	4	0	6
8	6	5	2	13
Total	40	12	4	56

Mean, all boys — 6.0 grades completed
S.D. — 1.4 grades

APTITUDES AND DISABILITIES—GENERAL

Health and Development

As far as could be ascertained, these boys were physically in good health, with sensorimotor development within normal limits, except for the one case of congenital partial deafness discussed below. No gross neurological abnormalities were observed, although the specific language disability symptoms themselves perhaps suggest what Critchley (1964) calls "minor neurological signs."[2] Confusions as to time, space or laterality, "nonspecific clumsiness," and other phenomena sometimes noted did not generally appear in medical reports of that period in connection with school age language problems, except in those by Orton and his colleagues. Some items in the Rose Valley histories might now be called "soft neurological signs." Data on birth, prematurity and perinatal injury were recorded in only a few cases, not enough to justify consideration here.

Some Sensory and Emotional Problems

The boy, already mentioned, who had a profound monaural deafness of congenital origin had very poor auditory attention and comprehension, vocabulary, reading comprehension, and verbal self-expression. His spelling, when visual learning predominated, seemed relatively good, as did his arithmetic. He was not classified as dyslexic, although he was given considerable tutorial help. In his secondary school a member of that staff spoke of a "reading disability, characterized by reversals." Perhaps the elementary school diagnosis was in error, but when young this boy showed a deficiency in basic language, and the deficiency seemed to derive from lack of

---

[2] Critchley says, on page 60, "In recapitulating the diverse neurological disorders which may be uncovered after close and particular scrutiny, it must be stressed that these findings are by no means integral. Many a dyslexic—perhaps even the majority of cases—show no such disabilities, despite the most alerted and scrupulous testing procedures. Perhaps they should be regarded as important epiphenomena—significant when they occur, but not essential in any consideration as to pathogenesis or aetiology. Furthermore the younger the subject the more likely it is that neurological signs will be found, while with older dyslexics the greater the likelihood of a negative clinical examination." (He is discussing children of school age and older.)

assimilated auditory language experience. He later graduated from a good college, did two years' graduate work in chemistry at a large university, holds a science-technology position in a government agency, and seems to have made a generally good adjustment.

In two instances, especially, relatively severe primary emotional problems with which the school was not equipped to cope interfered with adequate school learning. In one case, of a nondyslexic boy who has now earned the Ph.D. in science from a well-known university, there seemed no barrier to elementary school progress other than the emotional one. In the case of another boy, now a noncollege skilled workman, with good social and occupational adjustment, a severe language problem appeared to coexist with the emotional difficulty. This appraisal was made by a neuropsychiatrist.

If one knows children as well as we knew these children, one is tempted to say that emotional problems are the common lot of mankind, at least of American middle-class mankind. Only a few of these boys seemed entirely free of any continuing problems, but on the other hand seldom did the emotional problems appear to be the cause of learning failures. The emotional *effects* of learning problems, such as low self-esteem or personal and family tension, were much more apparent, as were the greater difficulties in language learning remediation when poor emotional adjustment was strongly evident. There was no question that the emotional tone of child, home, and school and the rapport with the special teacher were highly important in the learning situation and required thought and care.

Incidence of Language Learning Problems

What appears to be a relatively high incidence of dyslexia-related problems in this population probably comes primarily from the fineness-of-screen factor. That is, symptoms—quite real ones—are defined more inclusively here than by some investigators. Also the high incidence reported may arise from a more detailed knowledge of the individuals' backgrounds than is common among authors of many studies. It is in line with the writer's experience to question whether there is not much more irregularity in the development of "the last skill acquired" in human evolution (i.e., language) than has hitherto been widely recognized. Most people compensate for many of these irregularities or deficiencies with little conscious effort. Perhaps the deficiencies are Money's "sign[s] [which] might also be encountered . . . in the healthy," referred to earlier (p. 4). There is relatively little awareness on the part of most people of the possible relationship of such irregularities, or "unimportant idiosyncrasies," to disabling forms which language disability may take and which are more readily observed. Consequently, very careful questioning or observations may be necessary to uncover minor, but possibly related, language problems in other family members, an inquiry not commonly pursued as far as it has been here. Like other patterns which seem to emerge from the amassing of data, this one probably deserves continued investigation with the use of a computer, with its near-perfect memory and its capacity for quickly identifying obscure correlation patterns.

The family language histories of some of the boys in this study, one history including members of seven generations, cannot be lightly brushed aside even though much of the material is anecdotal. While some apparently reliable data are available, an adequate study of this question of familial or genetic etiology of language problems is beyond the scope of the present investigation. The evidence from studies other than this one also strongly indicates that some familial factor is often present in language disability. Attention is called to the work of S. T. Orton (1937), Hallgren (1950), Hermann (1959), Critchley (1964), and, most recently, Walker and Cole (1965), and Zerbin-Rüdin (1967), among others.

A student of the etiology of language disabilities must of course consider all possible factors, recognizing that in an individual instance there will commonly be several contributing ones. Among these, the genetic factor is perhaps least understood and least often given adequate recognition. Recognized, it may lead to management which will give the affected individual appropriate help from the beginning of his language development. He may well need such help as he begins to understand and produce spoken language, and at each later stage, as he masters the "second-order symbolization" of print and writing, and still later as he manipulates the symbols of higher mathematics and learns foreign languages.

Intellectual Capacities

While tested intelligence is only one aspect of development interesting to a child's mentors, it is a most important one when the focus is on the learning of traditional school subjects. Each of the boys included in this study was given one or more tests of intellectual capacity. Some had many and varied tests, generally at the school but in some instances at other facilities from which reports were available. However, each boy had at least one Binet test, and for the purposes of this study we report one Binet IQ figure for each. With the oldest boys, born 1924 through 1926, the Stanford Revision, 1916, was used. In 1938, when the new Terman Revision became available, all the boys still in the school were retested by the author and thereafter this instrument was used universally with students tested at the school. A few of the boys were tested only by outside examiners, but in these cases also the Binet of 1937 (or, in a few early cases, the 1916 form) was among the tests given. Where more than one Binet score was available, the highest was used, unless for some reason it seemed invalid. In fact, there were seldom significant differences in test scores of individuals; where such differences existed the higher score generally seemed the one more closely related to the carefully observed and otherwise tested aptitudes of the boy.

The reader's attention is called not only to the histogram (Fig. 2), but to the plotting of individual scores in relation to the Language Learning Facility Scale (Fig. 3, p. 33) which should be considered in connection with the IQ distribution and its significance. A fuller discussion of the Language Learning Facility Scale (on which nondyslexics and dyslexics are ranked in relation to the absence, presence, and severity of language disability symptoms) follows the discussion of the reliability of the IQ scores, although logically this is one of those unfortunate situations in which each topic should come before the other! In Chapter IV the IQ scores will be evaluated retrospectively in the light of the boys' later histories.

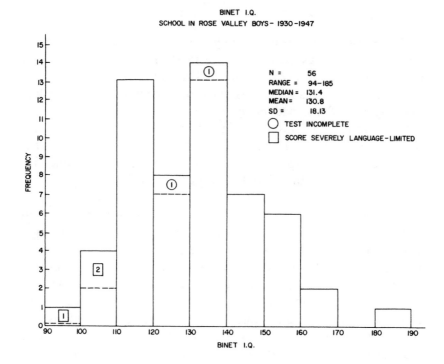

Figure 2. Binet IQ's—School in Rose Valley Boys, 1930–1947.

Reliability of the IQ Scores

Tests of two boys (given by another examiner) were discontinued before completion; the boys' IQ's of "at least" 136 and 127 were considered to underestimate their abilities appreciably. Since these boys were, respectively, Numbers 1 and 5 on the Language Facility Scale, the IQ's were considered to have minimal effect on the analysis of the data as a whole and were allowed to stand. The scatter of IQ's around the subgroup mean of the High and Medium Language Learning Facility groups of twenty and sixteen boys, respectively, was symmetrical, with no significant relation within the groups between Language Rank and IQ. *Within* the Low Language Learning Facility (or "dyslexic") group of twenty boys the visually noticeable association between language facility and measured intelligence was not significant. When the entire group of 56 was considered, however, the relationship between IQ and position on the language scale was significant at about the two per cent level, measured by either r (product-moment) or Rho (rank-order) correlation, a relationship which might have been increased slightly had the two incomplete tests been completed.

There were three cases (with IQ's of 94, 100 and 102) in which test scores seemed to be unreliable because of language factors. The partially deaf boy had a comparatively limited verbal understanding and use of words. While this was not judged to be a specific language disability comparable to those presented by his schoolmates, it did introduce a language limitation into his IQ score. His later history suggests strongly the probability that his innate intelligence was more truly in line with his brother's high score and his family's intellectual level, and was inadequately measured by the Binet test. The other two boys, who were Numbers 55 and 56 on the Language Learning Facility Scale, earned nonverbal (Carl "Hollow Square") intelligence test scores at the IQ 149 and 162 levels, respectively, at the time (with outside examiners) and one of

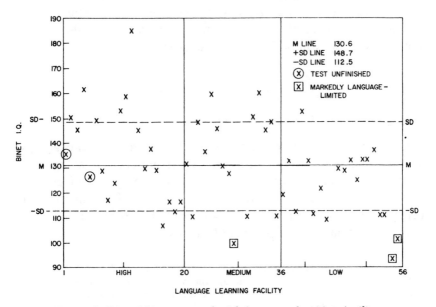

Figure 3. Binet IQ's compared with language learning facility.

them scored at the Very Superior level in adolescence on a Wechsler-Bellevue test. The later histories of both boys seemed also to bear out the judgments recorded by their examiners at the time that the Binet IQ's here shown were unreliable as measures of the boys' over-all intelligence. The lowest IQ of the series of fifty-six which the writer considers reliable is 107.

None of the twelve severely language-disabled boys, and only one of those considered moderately dyslexic, scored above 135. Yet all but two of these boys are now college graduates, several have doctorates or other advanced degrees, and one (*not* the 153 IQ) has earned two doctorates, Phi Beta Kappa, Sigma Xi and numerous other honors.

Apparently there were Binet IQ unreliabilities at the low end of the Language Scale which were unsuspected at the time of testing. IQ 130-135, in fact, seemed high to everyone concerned and there was little evidence recorded by the examiner that the boys were not functioning satisfactorily in the test situation. And so, while the Binet IQ is perhaps generally a satisfactory indicator, and far superior to most group tests where there are language difficulties, this study strongly suggests that even the Binet scale is a less accurate measure than we might wish when verbal problems are involved.[3] A retrospective study of matched pairs of dyslexic and nondyslexic boys will be found in Chapter IV.

LANGUAGE LEARNING FACILITY

Development of a Scale for Ranking

It was found virtually impossible to divide the boys into groups which could be clearly categorized by the presence or absence of language disability according to any criterion or group of criteria which would give sharply discriminative scores, either numerical or categorical. A scale on which the boys could be ranked on the basis of an evaluation of many pertinent factors was therefore devised.

[3] The Binet scales were the best available to the school at the time of testing, although the author now prefers to use the Wechsler Intelligence Scale for Children (WISC) with most children of seven or eight and older, especially if dyslexia is suspected.

Graded Series

There are at least two ways of getting a graded series of reading achievement or language learning facility or disability ratings of a group of subjects. One, which is common in educational appraisal, is to measure the learner's achievement against norms on a test battery and then, if it is appropriate to the investigator's purpose, to correct for intelligence level, educational opportunity, or some other factor(s). This might be called the survey method. Another, perhaps appropriately called diagnostic, uses the phenomena of language development and the symptoms of lag or disorder in the development of this function as its frame of reference. It then appraises the learners' achievements and shortcomings in terms of the presence, apparent severity, or absence of the symptoms and symptom clusters associated with specific language disorder, thus assessing degrees of facility in language learning. Many of the tests and normative scores used in the survey method are employed also in the diagnostic method.

Either approach could be used with a given school population as the basis for ranking the students in a graded series but the rank orders would differ somewhat. The first, or survey, method focuses primarily on the comparative effectiveness of the school in teaching, and the proficiency of the child in learning, language skills under the given circumstances. The diagnostic appraisal, on the other hand, is primarily concerned with identification of individual patterns of learning and their disorders as they appear in a given population and setting.

Reading (or other) deficiencies and proficiencies shown in a series resulting from the survey type of appraisal would include those depending on the full range of etiological factors, such as socioeconomic, educational and cultural opportunity, intellectual endowment, physical maturation, primary emotional disorders, and sensory and physiological efficiency, as well as specific language maturation. Such a series would have many uses in research and action. Whatever the etiologies involved, individuals would be placed on the basis of achievement, rate of progress, or whatever measures were chosen.

A diagnostic appraisal of a population, as here attempted, however, has a more restricted purpose. The full individual studies (from which this "diagnostically oriented" series was to be derived) were directed toward the discovery and remediation of any difficulties which existed, with attention not only to dyslexia but to any other factors of which the school staff was aware. Both developmental and remedial attention was given at the school to various aspects of growth and learning, many not included in this language appraisal scale, e.g., artistic talent or primary emotional disturbance.

The present study, however, concerns itself specifically with aspects of the language function, per se. Observations in considerable, though by no means exhaustive, detail showed wide variety in the language development patterns of the fifty-six boys here described. Some seemed to be "natural linguists" with no impediments to learning. Some had great difficulty; many were intermediate in ability to learn language skills. It seemed that the number and severity of symptoms of specific language disability (as here defined) was a fairly continuous variable which could be used to order subjects in a graded series which might facilitate the examination of the hypothesis being tested. *This hypothesis was focused not on the entire educational spectrum but on the problem of specific developmental language disability* as we had seen it in the childhood of some of the subjects, with their nondisabled schoolmates for comparison.

On this basis all the boys were placed in rank order on a continuum from what seemed to be the greatest (No. 1) to the least (No. 56) degree of language learning facility. This includes the learning of spoken language, reading, spelling and written expression skills in English. These ratings, as used in Figure 3 and Chapter IV, seem to be justified within the limits of the early data, in the light of the definition of specific language disability as given on page 4. It will be remembered that this definition is, in brief, the failure of an individual to achieve skill in one or more language areas, such as speaking, reading, spelling, penmanship and written expression, in harmony with expectations based on his age, physical condition, IQ (individual test) and educational opportunity.

The positional discriminations at the disabilty end of the lan-

guage scale devised for this study are probably better than those at
the facility end because more detailed data were recorded during the testing and diagnostic teaching of the boys who were having
trouble. At the lower end it is, by definition, a specific language disability or dyslexia scale. The whole ranking instrument *might* be
called a "dyslexia scale," but a more inclusive term was chosen,
*since all fifty-six boys were ranked and most were not categorized
as "dyslexic."*

It should be clearly understood that the boys were ranked only
on the basis of the factors related to specific language disability
or dyslexia, as here defined. There were, of course, some boys who
had academic inadequacies which seemed to result from such causes
as poor motivation per se, "late blooming," or generalized "unreadi-
ness" for academic learning. The placement of each of these boys on
the scale was determined not on such factors but on those directly
related to dyslexia (see symptoms listed on pp. 40–1), as well as
these could be isolated. Thereby the hazards of including "false positives" among the "dyslexics" were reduced if not entirely removed.

The language learning facility placement depended partly on
numerical evidence and partly on "clinical judgment." Many of the
records kept during the boys' elementary school years contained
numerical scores on standard tests. The qualitatively stated reports of regular and special teachers were also reviewed, with informal weighting based on many factors of curriculum and
teachers' personalities known to be involved, such as, "How pene-
trating were Mr. R's or Mrs. J's comments likely to be?" or, "What
factors in Edwin's school or home life, if any, caused Miss X to write
this report this way?" Experienced schoolmen and clinicians will
appreciate how much fuller the interpretation of such reports can be
when circumstances surrounding them are known. While most of
the information gathered was generated at the school, it was aug-
mented wherever possible by facts and opinions contributed by
physicians, psychologists and other professionally competent persons who had contact with the boys outside of school. Considerable
reliance on evaluative judgment was unavoidable, as the records
were not kept with a research design explicitly in mind, an inherent
limitation of this kind of *ex post facto* study. Every effort was
made, of course, to achieve objectivity.

Categorical Division

Where one divides "dyslexic" from "nondyslexic" in the present series depends on where the influence of the "dyslexic causality" begins to seem important in the language learning of these boys in this time and place. The divisions here used might not be those decided upon by other investigators. The findings with respect to the hypothesis would not be significantly affected however, were we to call only, let us say, the twelve lowest ranking boys dyslexic.[4] In fact, if one were attempting to "promote a cause," use of these twelve in contrast to the other forty-four might well strengthen the case, with their 5.6 years mean higher education, eleven bachelors degrees, six masters degrees and three doctorates earned by 1965.

The division made, however, includes in the "low twenty" only those whose childhood records show presence and/or severity of symptoms of specific language disability justifying, in the author's judgment, the categorizations of "moderate" or "severe" dyslexia. Recorded diagnostic evaluations other than the writer's contribute both to individual placements and to the whole matrix, as when a boy whose problems were evaluated only by the author was ranked in comparison with two or more other boys examined elsewhere.

This series of subjects, then, is ranked in accord with early records showing facility or disability in language learning in the framework of the writer's present understanding of developmental dyslexia.

Diagnostic Criteria

In general, difficulty with learning language skills was defined primarily as reading and spelling progress (or spelling alone in certain cases) inadequate to the school's standards. In the early grades, standards were determined more by amount of exposure to teaching than by grade placement. For example, when formal reading instruction was begun in second grade it was found that most boys and girls achieved one year's gain in scores by the end of the first year. They were, accordingly, not considered retarded readers if

---

[4] These "most dyslexic" boys are the ones who stand out, for example, in the matched-pair I.Q. study which was made later (see especially p. 93).

they were one year below *age* norms at the end of second grade, although their individual learning patterns might indicate the desirability of special teaching aimed at preventing problems. Normally pupils in regular classes made two years' reading gain in third grade and continued accelerated progress until reading proficiency approached mental age, which was the instructional goal. Eventually many children could be described with phrases such as "above grade 10.0 achievement at grade 6.9 placement," or "beyond twelfth grade scores at the end of eighth grade." Expectancies for spelling were lower, as: "Up to or above grade placement," or "Not markedly below other subjects" if the latter achievements were satisfactory.

Any child who seemed to need individualized help, for whatever reason, generally received it. However, in this retrospective diagnosis, boys whose problems were characterized by other phenomena than those generally associated with specific language disability, as described on pp. 40–1, were assigned to positions on the language facility-disability scale in terms only of the contribution of the dyslexia-related factors to their academic skill development, as far as possible. For example, the two "artists" (pp. 60–1), the boy from the bilingual home, and six boys who "bloomed" relatively late are scattered from positions 17 to 36. Of two boys with emotional problems severe enough to require their removal from the school, one (with high language ability and achievement) was rated in the high group of twenty, and one who concurrently showed massive language disability symptoms (diagnosed by a neuropsychiatrist) was rated in the low group of twenty. Boy No. 37 was judged to rate at the upper margin of the Low 20 group, although "late blooming" was a characteristic of boys and girls in his large "extended family" (known through two generations). He shared the "late blooming" characteristics of siblings, and other relatives but he was also "moderately dyslexic." Boy No. 36, with a very dyslexic younger brother not in the study population, was considered to be more a "late bloomer," although he had many specific language disability symptoms and responded to teaching appropriate to them. Perhaps the marginal boy No. 37 is a "false positive," although it does not seem so. There is perhaps as much evidence that boys No. 36, and those described in case vignettes No. 14 and No. 22 (see pp. 44, 45) are "false negatives." However, the adult accomplishments of the three being what they are, shifting the positions of these boys would not change the statistical picture substantially.

Certain **diagnostic criteria** were particularly important in the determination of placement on the Language Learning Facility Scale. The first consideration was generally *the initial failure of the boy to learn to read,* in the first year or two of reading instruction, up to the levels which were consistent with classmates' performance and his own general intelligence. The fifteen oldest boys began to have reading instruction at the school in first grade. The younger ones began in second grade. A few had their initial instruction elsewhere. Age at beginning reading does not seem to have made a difference in the boys' language classifications. There may have been some "critical period" factor, but it was not observable in the records.

The ways in which a boy failed to measure up in language achievement were important. His poor oral reading and word memory, the persistence of reversals of orientation and sequence, and the relation of inadequacies of skill in language to more satisfactory achievements in other areas were among them. Reading comprehension was seldom a problem in itself, but only as it resulted from failure to decode the written messages—to recognize or work out words and phrases.

The learning response to special language teaching often helped to distinguish the degree of a boy's difficulty. For instance, how hard was it for him to learn and retain phonics and blending techniques, important irregular words, and left-to-right sequences?

The persistence of characteristic spelling inadequacies was almost definitive of dyslexia. The boy's difficulty with analyzing words into component sounds, with mastering the details (as contrasted with the principle) of sound-symbol relationships, with letter orientation and sequences (such confusions as b-d, left-felt), with writing what he intended to write, with the superiority of copying skill over recall, and with breakdown of spelling in compositions, often to the point of bizarreness, were among the many problems noted. Scores in spelling, and also sometimes in arithmetic, where rote memory and manipulation of written symbols were factors, were often lower than scores for reading which these pupils had more or less mastered by graduation. Science, social studies, and mathematical understanding often brought higher ratings.

There were some additional problems. Early and even continuing *speech delays and inadequacies* such as late talking, misarticulation, stuttering, cluttering, etc., were more frequent among dyslexics. *Poor motor skill* in large and small muscle activities often called "dyspraxia" or "nonspecific clumsiness" was sometimes noted, as well as *poor penmanship* in those with otherwise adequate hand skills. *Verbal formulation* sometimes presented difficulty, as in word finding and immature syntax. There were some *auditory and visual perception and memory* problems, especially noticeable in sound discrimination faults when hearing itself was acute, and in recognizing and recalling forms of letters, numbers, and sequences in the absence of visual difficulties. *Lateral dominance and/or confusion* problems often showed themselves in the late or insecure choice of a master hand, and unsureness of left and right.

Many *family histories* contained reference to other members who had some of the above symptoms, not necessarily those presented by the boys, but these familial tendencies were not used in ranking for several reasons: the material was often anecdotal; this was not a genetic study; and some of the data lacked the requisite precision.

Each boy's language learning pattern was assessed individually, and the nature and degree of his difficulty was compared with those of the boys near him on the Language Learning Facility Scale before placement was finally decided upon.

The rationale for the choice of factors has already been discussed in an introductory way in Chapter I. More extended treatment will be found in S. T. Orton (1925, 1928, 1937), Gallagher (1948, 1960), Hermann (1959, 1964), Money (1962, 1966), Critchley (1964), Walker and Cole (1965), de Hirsch *et al.* (1966), J. L. Orton (1966b), and Thompson (1966), among others.

Table 9 shows the final separation of the fifty-six boys as rated on the Language Learning Facility Scale into three groups for purposes of comparison, and designated High, Medium, and Low. To recapitulate, the entire population forms a graded series, although the scale is not a numerical measure which is demonstrably continuous, but rather a close rank-ordering. The divisions are somewhat arbitrary, with individuals of very close similarity on both sides of the cut-off points, the low 20 being rated "dyslexic."

Table 9

LANGUAGE LEARNING FACILITY SCALE, 1930–1947

Category	Number of boys		Language rank identification
	Subgroup	Total	
High Language Facility Nondyslexic		20	No's. 1 through 20
Medium Language Facility Nondyslexic but with some symptoms of language difficulty	11		
Mildly dyslexic, clear but not crippling symptoms, individual help required	5ᵃ	16	No's. 21 through 36
Low Language Facility Moderately dyslexic	8		
Severely dyslexic	12ᵇ	20	No's. 37 through 56

ᵃ 1 case from this category and
ᵇ 4 cases from this category entered the school after Grade 1 because of its language re-education program.

The factor of birth order within his family was tested for each boy since this variable has often been considered important in psychological development. The proportion of boys in each language facility group standing in each sibling position proved to be strikingly similar, especially as between the High and Low groups, showing no apparent relationship ($\chi^2 = 3.81$, not significant) between sibling status and language learning facility (Table 10).

Table 10

BIRTH ORDER AND LANGUAGE LEARNING FACILITY RANK

Language learning facility rank

Sibling position	High		Medium		Low		Total	
	N	%	N	%	N	%	N	%
Only child	3	15	1	6	5	25	9	16
Oldest of 2 or more	10	50	7	44	8	40	25	45
Middle of 3 or more	3	15	3	19	3	15	9	16
Youngest of 2 or more	4	20	5	31	4	20	13	23
Totals	20	100	16	100	20	100	56	100

χ^2_{6df} 3.81 — Not significant.

Of the fifty-six boys, five came to the school because of its language program, four of them severe dyslexics. The other fifty-one can be considered linguistically "homegrown" (at the school). Of these fifty-one, eight or 15.7 per cent, were severely handicapped and the same number moderately so, making a total of 31.4 per cent incidence of marked language problems of a dyslexic nature. This is a high figure but not out of line with that found in some other populations. If the usual 4 to 1 ratio of boys to girls holds, the incidence percentages for the school as a whole would be just about the commonly quoted figures of ten per cent severely disabled and ten per cent more with handicaps severe enough to cause academic problems.

Eleven of the Low Language twenty, including ten of the lowest twelve rated severely dyslexic, were diagnosed "specific language disability" at the Institute of the Pennsylvania Hospital or elsewhere outside the school. In other cases a neuropsychiatrist at that Institute, Dr. Paul Dozier, served as a consultant. Clinical review of the author's diagnostic findings was obtained whenever possible.

Behind each statistic there is a person, and it is with these *persons,* whether indigenous to the school or "imported," that such a study as this concerns itself. In this case there are twenty boys who are called Low Language Learning Facility, or dyslexic, boys. They are compared with the other thirty-six, but especially with the twenty at the upper end of the scale.

VIGNETTES AND CASE REPORTS

Dyslexic Phenomena Among Nondyslexic Boys

Of the High Language Facility group of twenty, the first ten seemed to show not even minimal signs of language irregularity. Among the second ten there began to appear some indicators, minimal or transitory, such as history of delayed speech, somewhat poor spelling, penmanship of a character suggestive of dyslexia, or word-finding problems. In the next eleven, of the sixteen rated as Medium, such symptoms became more common, more noticeable and more persistent. Some of these boys were given tutorial help, although they were not considered dyslexics in retrospective diagnosis. The twenty-six boys from No. 11 through No. 36 are the subjects of the thumbnail sketches given in the "Case Vignettes" which follow. They are included to give the reader some idea of the scattered symptoms which seemed very prevalent in this population and quite possibly might be found on equally close examination of other groups. Following the vignettes will be found somewhat more detailed case studies and diagnostic notes.

Case Vignettes—Identified by Language Facility Rank Number

1–10. **No suggestion of specific language disability.**

11–20. **Considered nondyslexic.** Members of this group showed some slight symptoms. Minor shifts of rank might be possible, but mostly within the group. These would not be significant to the study's outcome, or if significant would reinforce its conclusions.

11. Slow to talk. Poor early articulation. Idiosyncratic vocabulary. Unexceptional penmanship. Extreme slowness in motion (not thought). No difficulty with reading, spelling, foreign languages, or the abstract symbols of mathematics. Brother "mild dyslexic—spelling." Several relatives with language problems.

12. Left-handed. Early penmanship poor. Scholastic record excellent in every field. Brothers "severe" and "mild" dyslexics. Several relatives, including son, with language problems.

13. No symptoms, self or family.

14. As an adult, still poor in spelling and penmanship. Excellent student in humanities, social science, biology. Brother "moderate" dyslexic. Other relatives with some language problem indications. On basis of follow-up data, either "false negative," or at least ranked too high on the scale.

15. "Slow starter" in reading and spelling. Good scholastic record. Cousin (in study) "severe" dyslexic.

16. No symptoms, self or family.

17. Poor school record, but from other causes. Home bilingual.

18. Early problems emotional. Excellent record later.

19. Artist. Difficulty with verbal formulation and expression.

20. Artist. Difficulty with verbal formulation and expression. Emotional problems.

21–31. **More pronounced symptoms, but still "nondyslexic" categorization.**

21. Poor motor coordination and control. Excellent student in humanities. Writer. In secondary school brother considered to have reading disability with persistent reversals.

22. In oldest class. Poor reader in childhood, still poor speller. Investigator's 1965 note after reading early records: "Although psychologist and teachers speak of 'emotional problems,' 'lack of confidence,' and 'immaturity' as causes of reading and spelling delay, I would now suspect dyslexia. Note high 'drive' and arithmetic success. Outside psychologist's recommendation of 'reading study' was not carried out. Further hindsight: boy repeated sixth grade in next school, but skipped most of twelfth grade, completed college in three years with summer school, winning two high honors and Dean's List citations. Binet (1916 form) at age 9 now thought to have been underestimate which unduly influenced our expectations of elementary school performance." Mother and sister reported themselves "poor spellers" in 1965. Boy rated in study as "late bloomer."

23. Family (the investigator was reminded by them in 1965) has always thought of this boy as "language disability boy, properly taught in elementary school." Ambidextrous, with poor penmanship containing many reversals. Excellent oral language. Reading not taught in first grade, no pressure in second grade. Teacher commented on his "understanding and deliberate control" of language learning problems in third grade. Accelerated one year in high school but then took postgraduate year in high school before college. No academic difficulties.

24. Early visual, motor and auditory problems. Some stuttering. First reading aptitude test rating "doubtful"; a year later "excellent." Late learning to tell time. Highly verbal. Brilliant academic record from end of fourth grade through graduate school.

25. Early and persistent speech problems, both stuttering and misarticulation, combined with precocious verbal formulation and oral expression. Several relatives with accepted or probable language problems, according to parents. Boy had no reading or spelling difficulties. Penmanship still poor. See "Walt's" case history, below.

26. Earliest reading suggested mild dyslexia. Responded quickly to minimum tutoring. Mathematics and spelling were still slightly below grade, much below intellectual capacity, at end of eighth grade. Spelling and penmanship still noticeably poor in adulthood, but he is a fluent and avid reader.

27. "Late starter." Some phonetically based tutoring; good progress. Remembered by the investigator as dyslexic, but the records do not show this. One of the youngest subjects, known by investigator only through mid-fourth grade.

28. Excessively slow-moving; perseverative. Many emotional problems, probably not dyslexic, although investigator never felt

quite sure. School learning problems continued, especially in written expression and foreign language, despite high intelligence. Reported to be an "A" student in philosophy in college.

29. In childhood partial deafness seemed to interfere with auditory attention and experience, language comprehension, and verbal formulation. Visual spelling and arithmetic adequate. Had general tutoring. Junior high school teacher said, "Reading disability, with reversals." (Such a boy might now be considered somewhat dysphasic.)

30 and 31. Brothers. "Late starters," perhaps mildly dyslexic. Older brother considered moderate dyslexic. All received and responded to, special language teaching.

32–36. Probably mildly dyslexic, Medium Language group.

If the writer were forced to dichotomize this entire population, she would be uncomfortable in not considering as dyslexics these five lowest ranking boys in the Medium Language Learning Facility group. Each of them showed more than one marked symptom of language difficulty and each seemed to need (and received) more individual help than those higher on the scale. And yet the response of four of them to special teaching was more rapid and "easier" than that of most of those lower on the scale. Perhaps the inner and spoken language facility reflected in their very high Binet scores was a factor here. One of the five came to the school in third grade partly in the hope of alleviation of language tension which had resulted in stuttering; he made rapid improvement. He read well enough, but needed help in spelling and certain aspects of mathematics. Perhaps he was not dyslexic, but a vivid picture remains in the writer's mind of an evening of family square dancing: this right-handed, well-coordinated boy, his moderately dyslexic, left-handed brother, and their right-handed father "swung" or "turned" their partners the wrong way most of the time, with a "dyslexic" kind of inconsistency. This is a striking instance of the fact that many dyslexics, not necessarily extreme cases, have difficulty in direction and sequence of bodily movements as well as in the manipulation of symbols seen and heard. M. W. Masland (1966 and personal communication) and others have suggested that the difficulty may be one of projecting a Gestalt as a model in space or time and then matching it in performance.

One of these five boys (the "Larry" of the third case study, below) read almost nothing until age eight, and then in a few months became a voracious reader. Another mastered reading with a minimum of special help. The spelling and penmanship of both boys responded much more slowly, despite their own and their teachers' continued efforts using special teaching methods appropriate for dyslexics. They went on to make excellent academic records, though in adulthood both felt hampered by spelling and penmanship problems of a character and severity which seemed like residuals of dyslexia. Another boy, from a family studded with dyslexics, needed more help in reading than did the two just mentioned and as much help in spelling, but by 1965 seemed finally to have mastered both subjects; he had always been a good penman.

The fifth boy in this group, No. 36 on the scale, had appeared to be another dyslexic youngster and for two years had been so taught. He seemed to be making steady, slightly accelerating progress when he left the school after fourth grade. At about this time an analysis by a knowledgeable diagnostician who did not, however, have the school records, found him "immature" and a "slow but careful phonetic reader," rather than what would now be called a dyslexic. He is here classified as borderline but *non*dyslexic, although the conviction behind this classification is not strong. The follow-up interview, in 1965, found him still an understanding but slow reader who had, by dint of hard work, made achievements typical of the other boys in the study, his field being scientific research. His younger brother was severely dyslexic.

These five boys taught the writer much about the value of early attention to relatively mild signs of difficulty. Whether each would have done as well without special teaching can not be known, of course.

37–56. The Dyslexic or Low Language Facility group.

The author has little or no question about the status of the 8 "moderate" and 12 "severe" dyslexics in the Low Language Facility group, except perhaps at the cutting points. The number and severity of their problems and the amount of extra help needed increases progressively with their language rank numbers. In addition to selected case studies, some individual symptomatology is reported as it is related to categorical placement, and the reader is also referred to the "matched pairs" study and to the family histories, both in Chapter IV. Although much evidence is available, only two case studies are given in this context because to do justice to symptomatology would make some individuals readily identifiable to others than themselves. We adhere to matters of "public record" in order to invade their privacy as little as possible.

Case Reports

Despite the statistical similarity of background and endowment, the boys as individuals are unique. No one of them can be said fully to typify his group on the Language Learning Facility Scale, no matter how unequivocally he belongs to that group. Still, a case study from each of the five subgroups may vivify their rather characteristic patterns.

The boys about whom much individualized biographical material is given in several parts of the study are comparable with one another. They are typical of the entire group in many important ways, and yet they do not describe the full range of variation. Some of this it seemed could best be shown in the brief notes of the case vignettes and some in the summaries following the Case Reports, especially the pages concerning the "other eighteen" dyslexics.

For the five case reports one boy each has been chosen from the first, or highest, group of twenty, the next eleven, and the following five, all thirty-six rated "nondyslexic." Of these, "Walt" and "Larry" have already been met briefly in the case vignettes. In addition, two boys were chosen from the clearly dyslexic group, one of them at the borderline between "moderate" and "severe" and the other somewhat more severely handicapped. The five boys are comparable as to background, intelligence, and subsequent history and achievement; they differ primarily on what might be called the "dyslexia dimension." All but one, who moved from the neighborhood at the end of fifth grade, spent their first six or more elementary school years at The School in Rose Valley. None of them is in the group covered in the Family Histories in Chapter IV. Additional factors in the choice of the two dyslexics were that each had been tested and diagnosed by a neuropsychiatrist and that, like two of the other three, the boy himself (not a relative only) had been interviewed in 1965. Each boy has seen his case history and assented to its use.

From the **clearly nondyslexic** group of twenty we have chosen a boy who will here be called *David*. (All names are, of course, fictitious.)

Dave had what his doctor would term an "uneventful" physical history except for a very mild case of polio when he was five, with no residual effects. His coordination was good and he "shone" at sports. He was "somewhat slow" in beginning to talk, his mother reported, and he stuttered occasionally at home and at school until he was seven. His oral language was otherwise excellent. His emotional and social adjustment were very good. His several intelligence test scores, earned both at the school and at a nearby university where he was seen periodically as a subject in a longitudinal research study, were consistently in the very superior to exceptional range.

He learned to read early and with little effort, "made his peace" with spelling which he found difficult at first. He says now that it has been "a vigilant truce rather than an absolute conquest." He developed a satisfactory manuscript handwriting which he still uses. He did well in mathematics, despite a professed dislike for the subject. Year-end tests from fourth grade on showed him above grade in all skill subjects. He was in the school from nursery school (age four) through eighth grade.

He made very good records in high school, college and medical school. He has published a number of scientific papers, is engaged in basic scientific research, and is working toward his second doctorate.

Other boys in the High Language group vary greatly in apparent endowment and in academic and occupational interests, histories and achievements. As nondyslexics they have in common that each progressed in language learning in a manner consistent with his endowment and his learning in other areas. None had language skill problems except as noted in the Case Vignettes, and when present these were minimal in their effects and in relationship to dyslexia.

Among the upper 11 of the **Medium Language Facility** group is *Walter.*

Walt had one serious language problem—speech. Both misarticulation and stuttering were extreme in early childhood, as observed before he entered nursery school at four. They persisted through the elementary school years, although there were only minor residual mispronunciations by the time he finished sixth grade. He was still stuttering occasionally then and in high school and is slightly hesitant in speech as an adult. His verbal thinking and capacity for abstraction were precocious, and his verbal humor, even in very early childhood, appeared to others as delightful, often even subtle—when his speech could be understood. There seemed to be no emotional cause for his speech difficulty, and few if any emotional effects of it. Home management of the problem was understanding and skillful.

Walt's handwriting was a quick and legible, but not neat, manuscript—a description which still fits. At first he was apparently right-handed and left-footed, and preferred the left eye for sighting; but by late childhood he developed almost consistent right-side preference. In this case it seems pertinent that there were at least five close relatives who had some dyslexic-like symptoms of varying severity (a fact verified by his parents in one of the follow-up interviews).

Walt's own speech difficulties did not interfere with his mastery of other language skills, for he became a fluent reader and a competent speller by the end of second grade (two years of instruction). Never outstanding at practical mathematics, he avoided the subject as far as possible. Still, he made good grades in this as he did in other subjects in secondary school, in college as a history major, and in graduate school, from which he holds a master's degree in business administration. He has a responsible position in business in which he uses mathematical thinking but not skills in calculation. He is active in civic affairs, including local politics and education.

Brief comments on *the other boys* in Walt's group of eleven will be found in the Case Vignettes. As in Dave's group, they vary widely, having in common the possession, at least in mild form, of one or more patterns similar to those found in more extreme degree or greater number in the "true" dyslexics. There may even have been one, or perhaps two, "false negatives" in this subgroup— boys who should have had more help than they were given with language skill development.

Larry has been chosen to represent the five boys who were categorized as **nondyslexic but closest to the dyslexia borderline.**

Larry, like Dave and Walt, had a very high Binet score. He was an early, fluent, and facile speaker and an eager listener, with an excellent oral vocabulary. When his group was introduced to reading in first grade, however, he was uninterested and apparently ·unready. When it was found that he really did not have reliable memory for visual word forms, instruction was not pressed and substitute activities were provided. Toward the end of second grade, near his eighth birthday, he "caught fire" and quickly became an omnivorous and understanding reader of anything which interested him, including many adult works from his grandfather's extensive library. If one were thinking only of reading, one would say that this boy, while a bit delayed in starting, was far from being a dyslexic.

But spelling, penmanship and the notational aspects of arithmetic were quite another story. Larry's visual memory, as is often true with dyslexic spellers, was adequate—more than adequate—for recognition of word forms where context, a large fund of information, and keen intelligence could substitute for exactness; but the recall of the letters in words, and the order of those letters, was most unreliable. Fine discrimination of auditory detail also gave him trouble. His large muscles were well co-ordinated, and he could do nice work with tools;

but when it came to writing, where fine muscles had to be used in the service of symbols, he again had trouble. The form of his letters was poor though his manuscript writing was legible. He often said letter names in one order when spelling, but simultaneously wrote them in another order. He understood arithmetic, but made many errors in written work. He seemed to be as free of emotional problems as any youngster in the school, and his motivation and attention were good. He worked hard during the special teaching sessions—half an hour a day for two years, in fourth and fifth grades. His was not a problem of hasty impatience or inattentiveness. By dint of hard, sustained effort, he raised his spelling and arithmetic computation scores almost to grade level by the end of the sixth grade, but his arithmetic reasoning was above grade and his scores based on reading and general information were outstanding. His written work, while excellent in content, continued to "look dyslexic" to one familiar with the signs of specific language disability in spelling and handwriting.

Larry did well in high school and college, although his grades might have profited from better spelling and penmanship, or he might have had to spend less time insuring their acceptable quality. His spelling, while it has improved, is still "undependable" and his handwriting has changed little in twenty years or more. Still, these difficulties apparently have not hampered him for he holds a very responsible position in the business world and engages in many activities, including membership on an elected suburban school board. He reads extensively for both recreation and profession.

Whether Larry is classified "dyslexic" or not seems to depend on where one draws lines of demarcation. As a reader he would not have qualified for the designation, except perhaps at first. As a speller he made progress with dyslexia-oriented remedial teaching, coming up four grades in achievement between the ends of third and fifth grades and holding the gain, though without further improvement, during the next, nontutoring, year. His difficulties persisted into adult life. Some language problems appear elsewhere on the family tree. For purposes of this study he was considered *nondyslexic*.

The other boys in Larry's small subgroup have been given attention in the summary following the Case Vignettes and three of them appear in the Family Histories in Chapter IV.

Henry and *Daniel* were chosen to represent the **dyslexic** boys.

Henry was unquestionably a member of the dyslexic group, on the borderline between a "moderate" and a "severe" classification; that is, just above the middle of the group of twenty. However, this is a rank —not absolute but relative to the other nineteen. We might as easily have chosen Garth or Harold or Roger further up in the "moderate" category. They had much in common, but Henry met *all* the qualifications for inclusion. He spent five elementary grade years at the school as well as a kindergarten year. His family was typical for the school and he for the 56 boys—at least on many statistical measures. His IQ was high for the dyslexic group (but at 29 points below his "match" in the IQ study [Chap. IV], it may well have been an underestimate). He was examined by a neuropsychiatric language specialist.

Because he was one of our early students, special language work did not get underway until his third grade year, at which point his reading was characterized as "rudimentary" (e.g., oral reading score —0). Our observations of the time: "Visual—short memory, reversals; auditory—good musical ear but inadequate speech sound associations; kinesthetic—speech gets tangled up, writing quality is poor and direction of making letters generally backward; laterality—right, after prolonged period of left and mixed; father ambidextrous; emotional—concerned over inadequacy." Until he began to succeed with reading he was a "red herring boy," always trying to distract the teacher's attention from the lesson program, but also wanting to stay beyond his scheduled lesson period "for more help."

The following notations were made in November of Henry's fifth grade year after two years of tutoring:

"Reading: Such tests as were given this Fall indicate that Henry has held his own in reading during the summer. Practically, we find that he reads with improving smoothness, accuracy, and assurance in a 4th reader. He is eager to try himself against a 5th reader, for which I think he will soon be ready.

"Speech: Most of Henry's difficulty with words up to 6 or 7 letters and 2 or 3 syllables has been overcome. With the longer ones he still has trouble with sound sequences and the insertion of extra sounds. It is easier than it once was for him permanently to correct his errors.

"Spelling: While Henry's spelling grade is very low 3rd grade, many of his mistakes in the shorter words are intelligent ones! On single words or words in lists he uses the phonetic knowledge which he acquired last year in reading, but makes wrong choices (e.g., spelling *nevir* for *never*). He makes many reversals and, in the dictation type of test, neither remembers a group of words nor holds the word he is writing well enough to apply the knowledge he has. His emotional attitudes and "escape" tactics are patterned exactly upon those which he used last year in the face of reading difficulty, though with greater force as the difficulty is greater and less easily mastered. However, we are giving systematic attention to spelling as well as to reading and hope for the same kind, if not the same amount, of progress here.

"Writing: Special attention is also being given and some progress made in making Henry master of his hand. At the moment writing is just one more high hurdle between thought and expression."

Shortly after this Henry was very thoroughly examined by our neuropsychiatrist and a long report was received: "Your diagnosis of specific language disability, or strephosymbolia, is absolutely verified . . . ," with special emphasis on sensory and motor normality except for the language function. The way in which Henry had responded to systematic, multisensory teaching was considered important. More tutoring time was advised and teaching suggestions were made.

A report for May of that third year of special work reads:

"Since Henry's visit to Dr. Dozier he has been having two half-hour periods of work daily and is making rapid strides in reading —is, in fact, practically up to grade, though not yet realizing his full possibilities. His handwriting is still extremely poor and a block to his progress in other lines but he has greater freedom of motion in the cursive script which he is now using than in the manuscript. Perhaps it is too much to expect form so soon. In speech he still becomes confused by some polysyllabic words but learns individual words much more willingly and quickly than he did. Only on the more difficult subject of spelling are the obstacles in the path of his keen, determined, and ambitious mind still sufficient to block his rapid progress. It is here that we are working hardest and must continue to work hard for some time."

At the end of the year his Stanford Achievement Test scores included the following, with the arithmetic computation score indicating a writing problem in his case:

	Grade
Grade Placement	5.9
Reading—Paragraph meaning	5.5
Word meaning	5.5
Spelling	4.1
Arithmetic Reasoning	6.7
Arithmetic Computation	5.2

At this point the family moved and Henry attended, for his sixth grade year, a rather conventional British school. He found the work very difficult at first, but by the end of the year he was "top student" in several of his classes and won prizes for achievement. Chance later brought the author into contact with one of his principal teachers who said, "I can scarcely believe Henry ever had trouble. He did at least as well as the others, often better than the best of them."

Henry became an honor student at one of New England's oldest and highest ranking preparatory schools, but found English and

French more difficult than mathematics and Latin. He graduated from a first-line university, earned a master's degree, and had completed most of the course work for his doctorate at the time of the follow-up interview.

He had worked in several business and public relations jobs and earned recognition for his writing (articles, not penmanship!). After successful employment as assistant to the managing director of a national trade association, he was just establishing a business for himself at the time of our interview and seemed to be setting it up with both imagination and acumen.

He reported reading slowly (but the books were substantial intellectual fare), spelling poorly, and writing legibly but not well—an example of successful adaptation rather than "cure" of dyslexia, and so not atypical.

Henry's daughter appeared in first and second grades to have reading problems not unlike Henry's own, but she has since become a good reader, speller, and penman. Her three brothers, one of them left-handed, all write poorly but are otherwise excellent students.

The second case history of a dyslexic is that of **Dan.** Dan had initially more severe problems than Henry because his spoken language was inadequate, although he had no difficulties of motor origin. His rating on intelligence tests was high for dyslexics (but seventeen points below his "match" in the recent IQ study). He entered the nursery school at four years of age and finished sixth grade at the School. He has at least two close relatives with histories of marked dyslexic problems. A few boys in the group had more severe problems than he had.

His early speech was full of misarticulations which continued at least until he was ten when, for example, he said very rapidly, "I wan'a new book—one what's recitene!" [rē-cī-tēn] A reading aptitude test at seven showed him at fourth percentile in articulation. Notes appended to his test read: "Weak on eye movements, sound blending, articulation, understanding of and memory for directions. . . . watch for reversals and fundamental confusions." An audiologist's test ruled out hearing loss; the problem was in auditory word-sound discrimination and memory, and in monitoring of speech. Reading, begun in second grade, proved very difficult for Dan, but he had persistence and determination and a very sturdy personality. He was given special help from third through fifth grade.

He, also, was examined by the neuropsychiatrist who had seen Henry, for consultation on the school's provisional diagnosis (confirmed) and for consultation on treatment. The speech, spelling and reading problems, the physician said, had their roots in auditory confusions of a "strephosymbolic" (dyslexic) nature. Poor visual memory for symbols was also a cause of difficulty. There were no sensory defects and Dan's motor skills (and his penmanship) were above average. He was sensitive about his problems and had a strong drive to master them and catch up with his classmates, two of whom had "graduated from tutoring." This kind of positively adaptive personality characteristic was noted in his nursery school record and observed in the follow-up interview more than thirty years later. A quotation from an early note by the author to the physician is illustrative: "Danny was given such impetus by his recent visit to you that he has forged ahead beyond our hopes. He was dissuaded from taking *Moby Dick* [standard edition] for the summer, not on the grounds of reading difficulty [his reading achievement grade at the time—5.0] but because he'd like it better year after next!" He was feeling hopeful about reading but spelling was still very difficult, as the following in-class composition from fifth grade shows:

"We had gests last night. Johnny Wang was from China. We had chicken, paes, and mashed potatoes. I helped to serve because we were late. and they were going in to see a dance recital. After everyone left I worked on my list of why poles are cold. I didn't know how to spell atmosphere. I spelled it 'apnasfear'. But it should be spelled atmosphere."

When he left the school after sixth grade Dan was a half year above grade in reading. He had a comfortable academic margin, but was still scoring below his mental age, in social studies and science. Arithmetic reasoning (as tested) was marginal; but scores in computation, spelling, literature, and language usage (despite excellent usage models at home and at school), were still below grade.

Dan, nevertheless, climbed to the honor roll and graduated *cum laude* from preparatory school. His records in a high-standard college and in a first-rank law school were excellent. He is now successfully practicing his profession as a partner in his law firm and taking active and responsible leadership in church and civic affairs. He continues to care intensely about people and to be greatly liked and respected by them.

Are there language disability residuals? His speech is clear and he speaks easily before many audiences. He most enjoys "books, food, and outdoor activity"—given in that order, with a grin. Still, he wishes he could read faster. He reported having learned to spell quite well, after continued effort. He had good English writing instruction in secondary school and college, and as Case Editor of the Law Review of his law school, he developed a logical, succinct, and polished style. The following is indicative of his adaptive approach: "I don't have a good memory for details but use reason instead. The law *is* based on reason, and so I generally come out with right answers, as I find when I check by looking them up in our law library."

The investigator's impression in 1965: "Sincere, rational, self-analytic. Prefers a calculatedly balanced way of life. Concerned with values. Socially responsible and active. Physically vigorous and, as always, full of good spontaneous fun."

In a recent letter, he said, in part, "I would be most willing to be Dan. Furthermore, I don't mind being identified . . . The only suggestion I would make is that you might indicate . . . that Dan went on to law school and is a practicing lawyer. This is a profession in which a good deal of attention is paid to language usage, and I think it might strengthen the point which you are making."

The other eighteen boys in the moderately and severely dyslexic groups all started in the school's first grade or preschool except the four who came because of their language needs; they entered the fourth, fifth (2) or sixth grades and stayed through the eighth. Of the fourteen who started in first grade, seven did not complete the school course. In one case parents withdrew a boy because of our insistence on outside diagnosis, and in another the boy was withdrawn as a result of our *not* having pressed the matter of referral! The other withdrawals were not related to dyslexia, except that one emotionally disturbed lad had both problems concurrently, in his neuropsychiatrist's opinion.

The two language learning subgroups of dyslexics presented a contrast—not marked at the division point—in the number and/or severity of dyslexic symptoms each boy presented. For example, only one of the moderate group of eight had a serious speech problem, but only three of the severe group of twelve had early histories *free* of such problems, and in most instances speech anomalies were still part of the grade school language pictures of these boys.

The moderates were all quite poor readers and spellers who needed considerable special teaching before they even approached competency. The lowest language group were all rated very deficient in both subjects and took longer to become independent readers. The levels of adequacy achieved at the school varied with the boys' length of enrollment and many other factors. Only one, a boy with severe language handicaps in several modalities, was not making much progress when he left the school after fourth grade. He and his parents persisted in their efforts to get help for him and he eventually succeeded, responding well in adolescence to much the same sort of training he was apparently unable to use in the early grades and later graduating from a university that had high standards. Progress in spelling was less satisfactory than in reading for all these boys (see Table 13, pp. 68–9, and accompanying text).

Low ratings in penmanship were neither uniformly present in the low group nor absent in the nondyslexic groups. Poor penmanship, it appears, may be a phenomenon in dyslexia, and when it is, the author's experience shows that the complications it adds to the life of a dyslexic speller are considerable (*vide* Henry). There were several boys in the Low Language group who shared Henry's unenviable lot—ten, in fact, for whom this poor penmanship was rated from a serious to a very serious problem. It is also possible that poor penmanship and poor speech in some cases are related to dyslexia in a broader sense without reading or spelling being involved. This view is unorthodox in relation to common definitions of dyslexia, but relatives of known dyslexics not infrequently present histories of speech difficulties (like Walt's) and/or show "a dyslexic kind of poor writing" as a major problem. People who work much in this field come to recognize the form and quality of such writing but find it hard to describe. Books on dyslexia, and my own files, however, contain many examples of such penmanship.

In addition to low scores and poor progress in reading and spelling, and prevalent but not universal speech and penmanship problems, the dyslexic group at The School in Rose Valley had more instances of poor motor functioning and more laterality and directionality problems than did the nondyslexics. The three boys lowest in rank all had extreme difficulty in these respects and lateral confusion was an exacerbating condition, if not a definitive one, in over half the Low Language cases. A sense of time and space and one's position in them was mentioned in two cases, one of them bizarre in its extremity: "One day I spent 'mos a whole day trying to 'member what my name was"—and when he entered the school at eleven years this boy could not tell time or give days or months in order. (Neurological tests showed no evidence of organic problems, and after some years his general functioning had become consistent with the higher fragments of his childhood behavior. By 1965 he was a very competent person in his early thirties, having successfully served in the army and having graduated from college.)

With these boys, such difficulties of "verbal formulation and expression" (as Henry Head phrased it with regard to aphasics) or "inner language" seemed to be a language problem, rather than one of general intelligence. The boy just referred to and three others in the low group had significant difficulty here. But then, so did the partially deaf boy and the two called "artists" in the comments on pp. 60–1. Perhaps this "inner language" difficulty should be considered part of dyslexia only when it is associated with other and more definitive phenomena. If extreme, such difficulties, however, might be called dysphasia, or might be misdiagnosed as mental retardation.

There were several symptoms which might have been expected but were *not* significantly present. In the school as a whole "drive," "motivation," and emotional tone were very good, and the Low Language boys pretty much shared this state of affairs. They sometimes became discouraged or, like Henry, used defensive or evasive devices but these were usually temporary. The problem of low self-concept was more prevalent and persistent among the boys who were diagnosed and given help *after* they had experienced failure, for then it was hard for them to believe that they were as capable and as likely to succeed as the accumulating evidence of their competence indicated. Low self-concept was, rather surprisingly, something of a general problem in this school, however. The writer has often encountered the problem in highly intelligent individuals whose life situations permit them to set their own standards. Perhaps they are bright enough to know what *could* be, but not experienced enough to accept human limitations. Bright children are vulnerable, especially in a school like Rose Valley where internalizing of goals, standards, and discipline is expected, and particularly if their language learning ability is at variance with their intelligence, for no one needs to point out their inadequacies: they are usually their own harshest judges.

Another phenomenon encountered only once, as a concurrent condition, in the Low Language group was generalized "late blooming." There were two marked cases and half a dozen less pronounced ones in the Medium and High Language groups where a youngster seemed generally immature but later caught up, apparently just with time and growth. While Larry was not included among the boys thought of as "late developers," *in reading only* he gives an example of what sometimes happens to a whole person when he seems to achieve a generalized "spurt" in maturation, catching up with his age mates or surpassing them as he fulfills his previously unrealized potentialities. Among the low language group, especially among the severely disabled boys, were several whose growth patterns fitted the "neurological maturational lag" concept of Bender and de Hirsch, but this seems to be of a different order from what is usually called "late blooming." The boys who "just seemed to grow up late" were excluded from the dyslexic group by design. They would have been the "false positives" for whom every investigator tries to be alert, but the "maturational lag" boys had many dyslexic symptoms.

Serious emotional problems, the kind that use up energy, or distort its flow into problem behavior, are also not in evidence in the Low Language group except in the two individuals who were *also* dyslexic. (One was graduated, one withdrawn.) Of course the school had its share of "difficult" children, and lived through difficult periods in the lives of many children, but only two of the entire fifty-six studied had to be dropped from the school because it could not cope with their emotional problem behavior. One of these boys was in the High and one in the Low Language group. Both were eventually rehabilitated and function well as adults.

On the whole, a summary of individual aspects of functioning of the twenty lowest ranking individuals, more or less typified by Henry and Dan, shows: close comparability of social background; a range of intellectual ability from average to superior; only two concurrent major emotional problems, with several minor or derivative ones; generally satisfactory, often superior, drive levels; delayed general achievement ("late blooming") *per se* ruled out. On the other hand "developmental or maturational lag" apparently related directly to language was common, as were laterality and directional confusion, mild motor inadequacies, poor penmanship, and mild to severe speech delays and anomalies. Poor early reading achievement was universal in this group by definition, as was the poor spelling which is even more definitive of dyslexia. Some motor, more auditory, and universal visual inadequacies in processing the symbolic forms of language seemed to underlie the conditions, although comprehension and thought (inner language) were generally adequate or better. A developmental lag in neurological functioning as it underlies language processes was postulated. Training designed in conformity with this postulate generally brought results—slowly, but to levels that permitted functioning which ranged from satisfactory to very superior.

An Aside on the Nature of Symbolic Expression

"The ability to construct by hand visually expressive artifacts often goes with inarticulateness, or at least the power to body forth makes words unnecessary," says Jacques Barzun in *The House of Intellect*.

To what extent should we try to fit academic ineptitude *vis à vis* "good intelligence" to a Procrustean bed of the dyslexic type of language disability? This problem may be partly illustrated by accounts of two boys who were verbally relatively inarticulate.

One boy, though he did not appear to be "an artistic genius," expressed himself better in music and painting than in words and numbers. His achievement test ratings in all subjects were low at the end of sixth grade, but spelling was higher than reading and both were above arithmetic, the opposite of the common dyslexic pattern. He was classified as nondyslexic. He completed secondary school without grade repetition, but gave up college after two years to take non-credit courses abroad. In 1965 he was reported to be working at a relatively low-level job, doing his "real living" after hours when he enjoyed the arts, including "writing, but not for publication."

In childhood the other boy, also rated nondyslexic, had more vigorous and dynamic use of artistic media at his command; he painted and acted as well for his years as the verbally facile boys read, spelled, and figured, in all of which areas he showed some inadequacies. In discussion of his very convincing artistic productions he was so completely at a loss for verbal explanation as perhaps even to suggest credibility for the theory that the artist is sometimes an unconscious channel for the expression in his work of "Truth" or "Reality"—or perhaps that his consciousness is of a different, nonverbal, order. At our recommendation this boy repeated one grade as he entered secondary school. He graduated from a college-level school of fine arts with a baccalaureate degree, and in 1965 was teaching part time in a similar institution, working as a designer, and enjoying the performing arts as his major recreational activity. He was reported to be relatively uninvolved with current events and world problems, although quite realistic about his practical and business affairs.

Perhaps it was not so much that these boys were "deficient in inner language" as that their individual capacity for expressing their quite adequate intelligence, and for relating to reality, was *symbolic* but not highly *verbal*. "Individual differences" they certainly showed; to say that they had "specific language disabilities" in the sense of the definition used in this book seems to the writer *not* justifiable. Boys with these kinds of verbal limitations were placed on the Language Learning Facility Scale in accordance with recorded judgments which showed something of the dyslexic or non-dyslexic nature of their *skill-learning* abilities in reading, spelling and penmanship in comparison with their otherwise demonstrated potential.

AMOUNT AND KINDS OF
SPECIAL LANGUAGE TEACHING

Early reading achievement was generally tested[5] by the use of Gray's Oral Reading Paragraphs, Haggerty Sigma I Silent Reading Test, Part Two, and the Iota Word Analysis Test, with others as trial or auxiliary tests, in addition to the classroom use of the appropriate Stanford Achievement Test Batteries. Spelling was tested by the Monroe adaptation of the Ayres Scale, Oral and Written, as well as Stanford and sometimes others. A variety of other tests from Monroe (especially those of auditory discrimination and sound-blending), Gates, and other sources contributed to each appraisal.

If it was decided that the child might improve his learning under the assumption that he had some form of the specific language dis-

[5] The tests used were Gray (undated); Haggerty (1929); Gates (an edition accompanying his book of 1935, not now available); and Monroe (1932) which contains in its Appendix, pp. 183–201, the Iota, modified Ayres Spelling Scale and other perennially useful diagnostic tests.

ability, the Orton approach came to be the strongly preferred one. Most of the special teaching was given in individual sessions. The boy was seen by his special language teacher daily, sometimes twice daily, for periods of fifteen minutes to one hour, depending on need and circumstances (Tables 11, 12). Records of lesson times are not accurate or complete enough for statistical treatment. Much use was made of library material; the use of "basal" readers was minimal. Both reading and spelling were stressed, with attention to speech and penmanship as needed. The keystone of work with the child was the mutual reinforcement and integration of the several

Table 11

SPECIAL LANGUAGE TRAINING OF STUDENTS — 1935–1947

School years of training		Number of students
None		21
<1.0	5	
1.0 — 1.9	4	
2.0 — 2.9	12	
3.0 — 3.9	12	
>4.0	2	
All special students		35
Total		56

Table 12

SUBJECTS TAUGHT BY SPECIAL METHODS, 1935–1947

Coverage	Students
One subject	5
Two subjects	27
Three or more	2
Other patterns	1
Total	35
Subjects taught[a]	Students
Reading	31
Spelling	29
Mathematics	5

[a] Penmanship included where needed (but often not as much as needed).

THE BOYS AT ELEMENTARY SCHOOL AGE   63

sensory avenues of learning, the exact procedure being varied to meet the staff's understanding of his individual needs.[6]

I was strongly influenced by Orton's statement (1928), "Our concept of strephosymbolia as a physiological variant rather than a general mental defect naturally gives a decidedly better prognosis, and there is not only good theoretical basis for the belief that the disability can be corrected and the children taught to read, but there is also to be derived from the theory a path of attack for such retraining." The spirit in which Orton's prescriptions were made and followed was summed up eighteen years later, just as this period at Rose Valley was coming to a close. "Whether or not our theory is right, I do not know, but I do know that the methods of retraining which we have derived from that viewpoint have worked. I do not claim them to be a panacea for reading troubles of all sorts, but I do feel that we understand the blockade which occurs so frequently in children with good minds and which results in the characteristic reading disability of the strephosymbolic type of childhood." (See J. L. Orton, 1966b, p. 265.)

The early teaching material, especially in the "Gillingham Manuals," made available a systematic presentation of the structure of the English language. It described methodical procedures for teaching by the simultaneous use of the senses of sight, hearing, and muscular awareness. But it was also adaptable in pace and detail to the individual needs and interests of the child, and to the ingenuity of the teacher who could use it as a base of operations to which other material could be added. It was an "approach," not a "method" or a "system."

Teaching with this approach is based on the teacher's integrating

---

[6] The pedagogical approach suggested and used by Orton in 1935–1947 was still being elaborated by Gillingham and Stillman (see their Manuals of 1936, 1940, and 1946). Further revisions in the 1956 and 1960 editions of Gillingham and Stillman, and in J. L. Orton (1964) improve but do not basically alter today the procedural approach used earlier. A review in some detail of both rationale and content of the approach that grew out of Orton's concepts and which are now used will be found in the chapter entitled, "The Orton-Gillingham Approach," by J. L. Orton in Money (1966). This is recommended reading for those who wish more details than can be given in the brief statement in the present volume about how the dyslexic boys in this study were taught.

his knowledge of the nature of the English language, and his understanding of the nature and growth of the language function in human beings.

The sounds of spoken English are graphically represented by the English alphabet. The correspondence between sounds and letters is not simple, but there are large and small patterns of dependability, linked together by logic and history.[7] Working familiarity with crucial elements of language (the phonemes and graphemes of the linguists) and their structured relationships gives the student operational power, with a rote memory burden limited in size so that it can be thoroughly mastered. Understanding of the system, at levels of sophistication appropriate to his growth, provides the learner both with interest and with a route for conscious storage and retrieval of needed linguistic data. Almost as a constant of symptomatology, automaticity, no matter how secure it may sometimes seem, is not fully dependable with dyslexics. The simultaneity of cognitive and stimulus-response learning allows the dyslexic more readily to "use his good thinking to rescue his poor memory," that is, to take advantage of that uniquely human aspect of his intelligence—the ability to use symbolic thinking to solve problems.

Neurology, neurophysiology, and neuropsychology in particular, offer valuable, if necessarily incomplete, understanding of the language function and its development in the learner. For the boys with whom we were concerned, learning to read and spell by establishment of exact memory of whole words was difficult in the extreme. The plight of such children had suggested to Orton the use of the smallest meaningful units of language (the phonemes of speech, and the phonograms or graphemes which are their written record), thoroughly learned and smoothly blended, as an economi-

[7] Examples: A *large* pattern—the pronunciation of the syllable before an added suffix is reliably indicated as containing a short accented vowel if the intervening consonant has been doubled, as in *hopping* or *beginning*. The reverse, as a spelling rule, is even more useful. This represents a large section of an even larger structural principle concerning vowel quantity, syllabication, and stress—part of the science of language which provides many dyslexics with an interesting route to greater security in decoding and encoding. A *small*, but useful, pattern—*ough* when followed by t is generally pronounced as in *ought, thought*, etc.

cal but sound and comprehensive strategy. These children had problems in one or more of the modalities used in language behavior—visual, auditory, and kinesthetic—and in the interrelationships of the modalities. If, therefore, the training made use of the student's simultaneous seeing, hearing, and awareness of muscular action while he made sounds and letters and their carefully blended sequences, there should result a solid foundation of skills on which to build language competence. The content of this training could not be randomly chosen nor casually taught; it had to be sequential and cumulative for each child if it was to be fully effective.

The argument raged then, as it still does, whether it was wiser to emphasize primarily what a child could do well, and so minimize failure and maximize the feeling of success; or whether one should attack vigorously those problem areas in which the learner showed the greater deficits, the ones which "needed overcoming." It was the author's conviction that one must do both—"strengthen the strengths" so that they could be depended upon to help in the areas of weakness, while the latter were being overcome as far as possible—with emphasis being given all the while to intermodal cooperation. "Sound it out while you trace it as you look; your ears and your muscles will help your eyes to get it—or to get it back if you've forgotten." "Say each letter name as you write it; now sound what you have written, to check yourself."

Development of scientific understanding and pedagogic skill in this approach in the 1930's and 1940's demanded even more exploration on the part of the teacher than it does today. Useful materials were hard to find, but suggestions for making one's own adaptations were available not only in Orton and Gillingham publications but in Akin (1913), Monroe (1932), Monroe and Backus (1937), Stanger and Donohue (1937), Fernald (1943), and in the standard reading textbooks of the day, such as Betts (1936) and Gates (1935).

The boys had varying needs—different areas of strengths and weaknesses, and differences in learning facility, often changing from day to day in the same child. The situation demanded flexibility as well as system and ingenuity, and also commitment to both the scholarly and the individual, or social casework, disciplines. These were necessary ingredients in the program that developed following the success of the early students in coping with their specific language disabilities.

Classroom teachers cooperated in the program, partly by tailoring their procedures to the needs of the children as far as was practicable, and partly by cheerfully excusing absence for individual sessions. The individual work was done either with the writer or with a succession of several tutor-trainees. No one thought the arrangements as nearly perfect nor the achievements as consistently good as ideally they might have been, but there was general agreement as to aim, genuine effort toward continued improvement, and a spirit of cooperation. Most of the students made gains which seemed satisfactory. Others appear to have laid the groundwork for later gain, even when their early progress was slower.

School Achievement Test Records

On the basis of test records and verbal reports of varying degrees of exactness, the investigator has attempted to assess the general level of competence of each boy at the time of his leaving the school, estimating the degree to which he had mastered reading, spelling and, where known, arithmetic. These estimates serve only as indicators (Table 13). One might point out further that by the time they left the school twenty-five per cent of the boys in the Low Language Facility group were reading at a superior level, forty per cent at a level close to their grade placement, and thirty-five per cent were still rated as inadequate by half a year or more, although most of them eventually learned to read more than satisfactorily. Half a year below grade at grade placement 3.9 to 8.9, which covers these cases, is not considered "retardation" in most studies, but stricter standards were used here. In spelling, however, only five per cent of the boys in the Low Language Facility group had reached the superior level, five per cent the average level, while ninety per cent were still below grade. Even though the numbers are small, this tends to fit with the findings of the Walker-Cole study (1965). But it is also true that the Medium Language group still had sixty-three per cent poor spellers and even the high group had twenty-five per cent who were not up to grade, something of a school-wide problem. As one might expect, the boys who stayed in the school through sixth grade or beyond, no matter when they started, showed better results relative to grade placement in their final tests than those who left before completing the sixth grade. Most of the "non-graduates" made up their deficiencies later, as we shall see in Chapter IV. The nature of the data so far analyzed does not justify further statistical treatment of these records at this time.

Table 13
READING, SPELLING, AND ARITHMETIC STATUS AT TIME OF LEAVING SCHOOL
(Last test, or teacher's assessment, not more than one year before leaving)

Groups	No. of Boys	Reading			Spelling			Arithmetic			
		I[a]	II[b]	III[c]	I[a]	II[b]	III[c]	I[a]	II[b]	III[c]	Unknown
High Language											
Grades completed ≥6	15	12	1	2	8	4	3	10	0	4	1
≤5	5	4	0	1	2	1	2	2	0	2	1
		16	1	3	10	5	5	12	0	6	2
% of 20		80	5	15	50	25	25	60	0	30	10
Medium Language											
Grades completed ≥6	12	8	3	1	1	4	7	6	5	1	
≤5	4	1	1	2	0	1	3	0	1	3	
		9	4	3	1	5	10	6	6	4	
% of 16		55	25	20	6	31	63	37.5	27.5	25	

68

Low Language

Grades completed	Total	I (Superior)	II (Average)	III (Inadequate)					
≥6	**12**	**5**	**5**	**2**	**10**	**1**	**5**	**5**	**1**
≤5	**8**	**0**	**3**	**5**	**8**	**1**	**1**	**5**	**1**
% of 20		*25*	*40*	*35*	*90*	*10*	*30*	*50*	*10*
Total	**56**	**30**	**13**	**13**	**33**	**20**	**12**	**20**	**4**
% of 56		*54*	*23*	*23*	*59*	*36*	*21*	*36*	*7*

Summary of grades completed

	Total	I	II	III					
All Ranks ≥6	**39**	**25**	**9**	**5**	**20**	**17**	**10**	**10**	**2**
% of 39		*64*	*23*	*13*	*51*	*44*	*26*	*26*	*5*
All Ranks ≤5	**17**	**5**	**4**	**8**	**13**	**3**	**2**	**10**	**2**
% of 17		*29*	*24*	*47*	*76*	*18*	*12*	*59*	*12*

a Superior, I — one year or more above grade — often much more.
b Average, II — one year above grade to ½ year below.
c Inadequate, III — More than ½ year below grade.

Note: Material in the foregoing close-packed table can be interpreted readily in this manner—note bold-face figures in the Low Language-Reading section which can be read as follows: Of the twenty Low Language boys eight, or 40 per cent, were reading between .5 grade below and 1.0 grade above grade placement at or near the time of school leaving; three of these boys left at or before the end of fifth grade, five of them finished sixth grade or more.

Chapter IV

THEIR ADULT ACCOMPLISHMENTS, 1964–1965

Sources of Information

In 1964–1965 it was possible to obtain current information about every one of the 56 boys who qualified for inclusion in the study. Twenty-one of the boys themselves were available for interview. Parents, siblings or other close relatives supplied information about those who were geographically inaccessible. In only four cases was it necessary to rely on nonrelatives, and in these instances each informant had had recent contact with the boy. (For example, one friend, an uncle-by-courtesy, had seen a boy in Florida just the week before the interview here reported.) In no case was it necessary to resort to correspondence alone. For some boys there were, obviously, two or more informants (Table 14). Wives of the boys participated with them in all or parts of several interviews.

Table 14

INFORMANTS, 1964–1965 STUDY OF 56 FORMER STUDENTS

Informants		Number
Subject, himself		21
Relatives		
Parents	36	
Siblings	10	
Other relatives	7	
All relatives		53
Unrelated persons		12
Total interviews		86

The major facts—those bearing on the hypotheses—as well as most of the other information reported are well authenticated, although information supplied by others than the subjects may lack detail which the boys themselves could have supplied, and may even contain minor inadvertent inaccuracies, as in the case mentioned below. If time and funds had permitted, each of the boys would have been seen in person; such additional interviews are still being held as opportunity affords. For example, during the manuscript preparation one moderately dyslexic boy brought his severely dyslexic daughter to me for testing. Three other boys, including "Walt" of Case History 2, were also interviewed when unrelated objectives took me to the Pacific Coast.

Almost all respondents were cordial and helpful; most, including all of the boys, were enthusiastically interested. In one case of a relatively low achieving, nondyslexic, geographically distant boy, the father, who was of professional status, was brusque, refused a personal interview, but gave all the necessary and some incidental information over the telephone. The reluctance of this cooperation was most atypical.

Much information was culled from the school files, including the two previous follow-up questionnaire studies. The writer, having long had in mind some sort of "longitudinal study of ex-nonreaders," had also kept a file of information about some of the boys for many years. Most of the data presented in this chapter, however, were freshly gathered.

The interviews with respondents were carried out informally, but with a printed schedule in hand. Some questions were direct and factual. "When did [you/he] graduate from high school?" "Did [you/he] repeat or skip any grades?" Others, asking for judgment, opinion or feeling, were general or open-end in form. "How much reading do you get done nowadays?" "What sorts of reading material do you find interesting?" Do you consider yourself a fast, average, or slow-speed reader?" "Have you ever timed your reading speed?" "Do you enjoy reading, or do it only for utilitarian reasons?" In some cases there were such jocularities as, "When would you say you licked the spelling problem?" To that a respondent whose writing now seldom contains a misspelled word, answered, "You must be kidding. The dictionary is the most dog-eared book on my desk!" His mother, interviewed earlier, had thought of him as "a good speller now." This mixture of specific and open-end questioning was undertaken not without plan but deliberately, to elicit the maximum participation and information within the limits set by resources of time and skill, and to maintain conditions of rapport which were natural and sincere. The aim was what someone has called, "The integration of empathy and discipline on the interviewer's part."

Ages of Subjects at Time of Follow-up

In 1964–1965 the oldest boys were forty years of age and the youngest were twenty-six. The mean age of the group was 33.4 years, with a standard deviation of 3.5 years; the median age was 34.4 years. The relationship of age to several other variables was examined, the older half of the population being divided from the younger half for this purpose on the basis of actual birth dates.

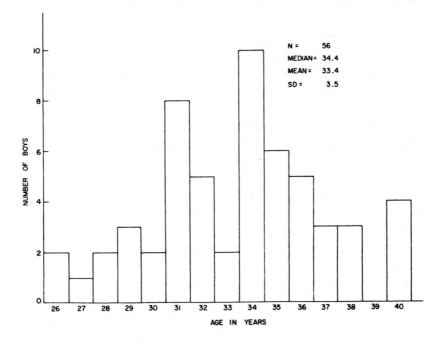

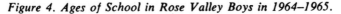

Figure 4. Ages of School in Rose Valley Boys in 1964–1965.

One boy had died two years before the 1964–1965 study began, but since he had completed his schooling and was established in his profession at the time of his death, the facts about him are reported with those pertaining to his forty-year-old classmates. This boy was, by a month, the oldest subject in the study, the one whose language difficulties had led to the establishment of the school's diagnostic and remedial program, and to whom this monograph is dedicated.

ADULT ACHIEVEMENT—EDUCATION

After they left The School in Rose Valley most of the boys made steady progress through secondary school, with promotion each year and high school graduation at about age eighteen. In a few cases there were accelerations of a year or loss of grade of a year, or some other irregular pattern, but the number of such instances was not large enough for statistical treatment. Grade repetitions were reported for three severe and two moderate dyslexics. Two of these five boys were among those who had not graduated from college by 1965. While it was scholastic inadequacy, not necessarily of dyslexic origin, which sometimes necessitated grade repetition, some boys went on from The School in Rose Valley to independent (i.e., private) schools with twelve-year programs where the policy was almost invariably to require entering transfer students to repeat one grade.

By 1964–1965 all the boys were high or college preparatory school graduates and forty-eight of the fifty-six had earned at least their baccalaureate degrees, with three others still enrolled as undergraduate degree candidates. All fifty-six had pursued some sort of further training beyond secondary school, all but one having had some college experience (Tables 3 and 4, Chapter III; Figures 5 and 6, and Tables 15, 16 and 17). Education is reported in terms of years of schooling completed, not calendar or school years attendance.

The mean number of years of post-high school education achieved by the boys was 5.73, with a standard deviation of 2.15 years. There was a striking similarity of these figures with those describing the fathers' attainment (M. 5.84, S.D. 2.17). A comparison of older and younger boys shows the older twenty-eight boys to have achieved

Table 15
YEARS OF HIGHER EDUCATION OF 56 BOYS, 1964–1965,
AND OF THEIR FATHERS, 1930–1947

Years of higher education	Boys	Fathers[a]
0	0	1[b]
1	1	0
2	1	1
3	5	0
4	14[c]	19
5	7	0
6	5	8
7	8	11
8	12	16
9	0	0
10	2	0
11	1	0
Totals	56	56
Mean in years	5.73	5.84
S.D.	2.15	2.17

Differences not significant

[a] Parents are counted once for each boy. See Note, Table 3.
[b] Calculated as −4 years, no high school.
[c] One not college graduate; equivalence based upon one year in college and four and a half years in technical school.

0.61 of a year more of schooling than had the younger twenty-eight, which is not statistically significant. It is interesting to note that the ages of the boys in each Language Facility group were symmetrically ranged around the group mean age, which in turn was in each case very close to the population mean. There was, for example, a difference of only .34 years between the mean age of the population and that of the Low Language Facility group. Year of birth does not seem to have contributed to language learning facility in this population, which should be no cause for surprise.

The surprise comes when we examine the mean number of college and university "years' worth" of higher education completed by each of the Language Learning Facility groups and find these to be 5.45, 5.69 and 6.02 years for the High, Medium and Low groups, respectively, in that unexpected order of magnitude. The differences (in terms of trend of means) are not large enough to have statistical significance, but the direction of difference seems at least noteworthy. In general, members of the Low Language Facility group have not been enough hampered by the residual effects of dyslexia to prevent their attaining schooling about equivalent to that required for a master's degree each.

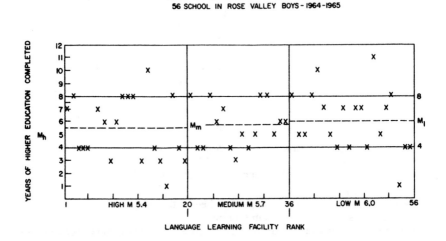

Figure 5. Years of higher education completed by 1964–1965, compared with language learning facility. (See also Table 16.)

A closer look at individual records of the twenty boys adjudged dyslexic in childhood shows two boys who were not college graduates; four who had by 1964–1965 achieved bachelor's degrees only; four who had each added one year of graduate study; one who had a law degree, one a graduate degree in divinity, and three others, already with master's degrees, who were doctoral candidates; five already with doctorates, one of them with two years' post-doctoral study and another with a Ph.D. in addition to his M.D. This seems, indeed, an encouragingly good record to have been made by a group of true dyslexics, some of them with severe initial handicaps. Could one conjecture that a disability, when it is not insuperable, may act as a spur to achievement? Some research in motivation and learning points in that direction [Berlyne (1966)].

Table 16

HIGHER EDUCATION OF BOYS IN THREE LANGUAGE FACILITY
GROUPS, 1964-1965

School Years of Higher Education[a]	High 20	Medium 16	Low 20	Total
1	1	0	0	1
2	0	0	1[c]	1
3	4	1	0	5
4	5	4	5[b]	14
5	0	3	4	7
6	2	3	0	5
7	2	1	5	8
8	5	4	3	12
9	0	0	0	0
10	1	0	1	2
11	0	0	1	1
Totals	20	16	20	56
Mean years higher education	5.45	5.69	6.02	5.73
S.D.	2.37	1.64	2.39	2.15
$t_{trend\ of\ means}$	1.07 — not significant			

[a] Degree year equivalences: Bachelor's—4; Master's—6; Law—7; MD, PhD, JD, ScD—8; 2nd doctorate—11; internship and residency ignored.
[b] One not college graduate; equivalence based upon college and technical school.
[c] Equivalence based on technical school only.

While some of the boys' university study is probably a result of the availability of "G.I. Bill" (veterans' education) funds, there is no evidence that this influence was appreciably greater in one language group than another. On a case basis we observe that two of the three boys (all nondyslexics), still supporting themselves while enrolled as undergraduates, are nonveterans.

Questions may be raised as to whether or not the dyslexic boys achieved their rather surprising record by "choosing easy colleges" and whether they could repeat the achievement if they were going to school in the 1960's. While there is some variation in the admission requirements and difficulty of colleges chosen, the list of institutions from which the boys received undergraduate and graduate degrees (Table 18) says "No" to the first question and suggests an answer to the second. While the boys might have more trouble gaining admission to the colleges of their first choice today, the institutions most of them attended already had highly selective ad-

Table 17
HIGHER EDUCATION OF 28 OLDER AND 28 YOUNGER BOYS, 1964–65

Years Higher education[a]	Older Half	Younger Half	Total
1	1	0	1
2	1	0	1
3	2	3	5
4	4	10	14
5	3	4	7
6	3	2	5
7	5	3	8
8	7	5	12
9	0	0	0
10	1	1	2
11	1	0	1
Totals	28	28	56
Mean years higher education	6.04	5.43	5.73
S.D.	1.69	1.52	2.15
Diff. of means		0.61	
χ^2		not significant	

[a] Degree year equivalences: Bachelor's—4; Master's—6; Law—7; MD, PhD, JD, ScD—8; 2nd doctorate—11; internship and residency ignored.

EDUCATIONAL ACHIEVEMENT – AGE RANK
56 SCHOOL IN ROSE VALLEY BOYS – 1964–1965

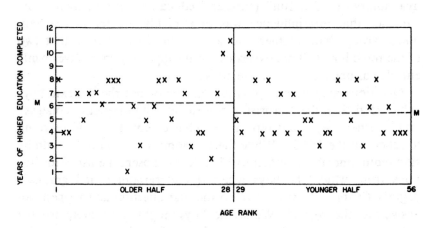

Figure 6. *Years of higher education completed by 1964–1965, compared with age rank. (See also Table 17.)*

mission policies and exacting standards of scholarship even in the 1940's and 1950's.

Table 18

INSTITUTIONS OF HIGHER LEARNING GRANTING DEGREES
TO 18 BOYS IN LOW LANGUAGE GROUP

Undergraduate	No. Degrees	Graduate	No. Degrees
Haverford	4	University of Pennsylvania	6
Swarthmore	3	Boston University	1
Brown	1	Columbia	1
Connecticut Wesleyan	1	Harvard	1
Cornell	1	Michigan State	1
Earlham	1	N.Y. University	1
Lafayette	1	Temple	1
Oberlin	1	University of Wisconsin	1
Pennsylvania Military College	1	Yale	1
Temple	1	Total	14
University of Pennsylvania	1		
Williams	1		
Yale	1		
Total	18		

OCCUPATIONAL ACHIEVEMENT

In 1964–1965 all the boys were employed, including those who were also college or university degree candidates.

Table 4, Chapter III, has shown the variety of occupations followed by the group as a whole.

These occupations were classified as closely as was possible in accordance with the scale given in Warner's *Social Class in America*, (1949, pp. 140-141). This scheme was used in assigning a socioeconomic class rank to each boy. A score of 1.0 was assigned to Class I, professional or higher business; 2.0 to Class II, subprofessional or middle business; 3.0 to Class III, minor business; 4.0 to Class IV, factory foreman or worker in skilled trades; 5.0 to Class V which includes skilled workers still in training and those in "medium skill" occupations. This, of course, meant that the higher status positions carried the lower numerical scores. These classifications are shown in Table 19 for the Language Learning Facility groups and the Age groups.

Table 19
SOCIOECONOMIC STATUS OF 56 BOYS, 1964–65, BY
LANGUAGE FACILITY AND AGE GROUPS

Language Facility Group	Socioeconomic Class							
	I	II	III	IV	V	Total	Mean ±	S.D.
High	9	6	4	0	1	20	1.90	1.19
Medium	6	7	3	0	0	16	1.81	.72
Low	9	9	0	1	1	20	1.80	1.12
Total	24	22	7	1	2	56	1.84	.96
Age Group								
Older	16	6	3	1	2	28	1.82	1.20
Younger	8	16	4	0	0	28	1.86	.63
Total	24	22	7	1	2	56	1.84	.96

The older boys were found to be very slightly ahead of the younger boys in socioeconomic status. Some interesting details of the age related differences will be discussed in connection with age and generation patterns in achievement. With the Language Facility groups the order of relative magnitude found for educational achievement repeated itself on the occupational scale. The Low Language Facility group had the highest rating; the differences were slight but the direction was unexpected. To the roster of occupations the Low Language Facility group of boys contributed the following:

Doctor (Medical)	2	(both research scientists and one also a Ph.D. in bio-chemistry and a college professor)
Lawyer	1	(partner in firm)
College professor	2	(one a department head)
Research scientist	2	(other than medical)
Owner medium business	3	(one also had minor level business job)
"Middle management" (jr. business exec.)	3	
School principal	1	
Secondary school teacher, MA	1	
Secondary school teacher, BA	2	
Actor (regular, contract)	1	
Factory foreman	1	
Skilled laborer — in training	1	

(If the five boys thought "mildly dyslexic" had been included this would have added three more research scientists, one of them also a college professor and one a college instructor, as well as one upper- and one middle-management businessman.)

EXAMINATION OF HYPOTHESES

Although other material which may throw interesting light on similarities and differences within the school population has been analyzed and will be found below, evidence which bears directly on the stated hypotheses is now before the reader. It is summed up in Figure 5 and Tables 16 and 19, and in the accompanying text.

Null Hypothesis

The hypothesis in the null form, as stated in the Introduction, must be accepted for the population under study. This hypothesis reads, "Given average or better intelligence, physical normality, and equivalent social and educational opportunity in both groups, differences in educational and vocational achievement by adulthood on the part of nondyslexic boys, and dyslexic boys so diagnosed between the ages of six and twelve, will not be greater than could be explained by chance alone." On the basis of the data presented this seems clearly to be an acceptable conclusion.

Clinical Hypothesis

On the other hand, the clinician's hypothesis must be rejected. This hypothesis as posed by the clinician was oppositely, and more simply, stated: "Dyslexic students, so diagnosed between the ages of six and twelve, necessarily have substantially poorer prospects than do nondyslexic students for success in later educational and occupational achievement." Clearly, on the basis of the same evidence, this hypothesis is not acceptable. In fact, the small differences which have occurred thus far in the group here studied, while statistically nonsignificant, nevertheless favor the dyslexic boys noticeably on the measures of education and slightly in occupational achievement. Conservatively one can say that *these* dyslexics have made at least as good records as their nondyslexic fellows.

Of course, this by no means proves, or even suggests, that *all* dyslexics are *good* academic and occupational risks, but the evidence clearly shows that dyslexics cannot be judged to be *poor* risks on the basis of language disability alone; this should be considered when prognoses are being made. Advice to keep the educational and occupational sights very modest would have been inappropriate for most of these boys and it accords with much of the less systematically analyzed experience of the writer and others that this is true for many dyslexics of otherwise high potential.

AGE, GENERATION AND ACHIEVEMENT

Reasons for the Study of Age Factors

The variations in achievement related to the ages of the boys in 1964–1965 and to the age and/or culture differences between the boys and their fathers seemed worthy of examination for three reasons.

In the first place, in this relatively small group there might have been some fortuitous connection between age and Language Learning Facility rank which would falsely negate or exaggerate the similarities or differences among the language learning facility groups with respect to the critical measures of educational and occupational achievement. For example, there might have been shifts in the character of the school's constituency with regard to socioeconomic status, cultural expectations, or language learning ability, either on a chance basis or because of school policy, community changes, or for unknown reasons.

Secondly, even if this sort of connection were ruled out with this group, it might still operate in comparable studies whose authors might find interesting and useful the data and methods of analysis reported here.

Thirdly, since this study had concerned itself with the sociology of its population as a whole as background for the understanding of the specific problem, the data on ages and generations seemed pertinent.

As has been said, in the three Language Learning Facility groups the mean ages were found to cluster closely about the population mean; the Older and Younger groups were almost equally represented in each Language Learning Facility group. Age, then, was not a determiner of language rank in this population, but it did seem to have some relation to the vocational achievements measured among the boys, and perhaps of the boys compared with their fathers.

Education of Fathers and Sons

Reference to Table 15 will quickly demonstrate the near equality in the amount of schooling of the boys and of their fathers. While most of the boys had finished most of their formal education by the time the data recording was completed in 1965, several were still candidates for undergraduate or advanced degrees. Two additional advanced degrees had been reported by the time the manuscript for this monograph was being prepared and there will doubtless be a few others, so that in time the boys' average academic education will increase slightly and probably equal or perhaps exceed their fathers'.

In the light of changing patterns of education for the professions, the exact significance of the comparison of the generations is not entirely clear. On the average the boys "equal" their fathers' achievement, but perhaps in the 1960's the expectations in the professions require more schooling. In this group of 56 boys, for example, postdoctoral university education is being reported where it was all but unheard of a generation ago. To be sure, individual study—"lifelong education"—was common with these parents, as it is with their sons. The intellectual "life styles" of the two generations probably differ less than the use they make of institutional facilities for keeping abreast of the fields of knowledge in their respective disciplines.

One boy, "David" of the case histories, has recently written, ". . . As you are undoubtedly aware, the fields of biochemistry and physiology have, in general, reached a level of sophistication which requires that those contemplating [university] teaching and research must undergo training beyond the introductory courses given in medical school. My choice lay between informal and formal instruction. For several reasons I chose the formal training program which I am now about half way through." Three of the boys who have M.D.'s and are in research have, or will have, second doctorates. Neither of the two M.D. fathers follows this pattern.

Socioeconomic Status of Fathers and Sons

A comparison of the boys' occupational achievements with those of their fathers proved interesting (Tables 20 and 21). All socioeconomic ratings were scored as before (see Table 19 and text), that is, to say, the higher the status the lower the numerical score in these ratings. Among the boys, the Older and Low and Medium Language Facility groups, at 1.82, 1.80, and 1.81 respectively, ranked very slightly better in vocational achievement than the population average of 1.84. The Younger and High Language Facility groups, at 1.86 and 1.90 rated a little lower but these differences were all statistically nonsignificant.

Table 20

SOCIOECONOMIC CLASS OF 56 BOYS IN 1964–1965, AND OF THEIR FATHERS IN 1930–1947

Status	Number of Boys	Their Fathers
Class I	24	46
Class II	22	5
Class III	7	4
Class IV	1	1
Class V	2	0
Totals	56	56
Mean	1.84[a]	1.29[a]
S.D.	.96	.66
Difference in means	.55	
t[b] 110 d.f.	3.5	

[a] Using the scoring standards discussed in connection with Table 19.
[b] t determined as if each column had 56 values — $P < .01$ ($.01 = 2.58$).

In contrast, the picture presented by the fathers was substantially different from that of the boys in every classification (Tables 20 and 21). The mean for all fathers was 1.29 (fathers counted as 56, one for each boy, see Chapter III). While detailed information was not available as to shift of status while their sons were in elementary school, the writer, who knew most of these families well, was aware of only a few such changes. The fact that the fathers of the older

Table 21

AVERAGE SOCIOECONOMIC STATUS OF BOYS IN 1964-1965,
AND OF THEIR FATHERS IN 1930-1947 — IN THREE
LANGUAGE FACILITY GROUPS AND TWO AGE GROUPS

Language Learning Facility Groups	Mean ratings ± 1 S.D.		Differences of Means
	Boys	Fathers	
High	1.90 ± 1.19	1.20 ± .51	.70
Medium	1.81 ± .72	1.38 ± .70	.43
Low	1.80 ± 1.12	1.30 ± .78	.50
Age Groups			
Older	1.82 ± 1.20[a]	1.18 ± .54	.64
Younger	1.86 ± .63[a]	1.39 ± .82	.47
Total	1.84 ± .96	1.29 ± .66	.55[b]

[a] Analysis of variance shows difference in S.D's. significant beyond .01 level.
[b] t test significance beyond .01 level (see Table 20).

group, rated at 1.18, were of somewhat higher status, on the average, than the fathers of the younger group at 1.39, may or may not be important. Since each father appears with each son, eight fathers are rated twice and two are counted three times, some in both age groups; as it happens, this introduces less bias than one might expect, but still too much should not be asked of the figures. The scores of the fathers are useful here primarily as descriptive background for the fifty-six boys, rather than for analysis of the fathers as a group of forty-four men, which is not the purpose of this study. Still for whatever it may be worth, we may note that the difference between the ratings of the fifty-six boys and the "fifty-six fathers" achieves a statistical significance beyond the .01 level.

Age and Occupational Achievement Among the Boys

The standard deviations of the distribution of each subgroup's socioeconomic scores is noticeably larger for the older boys and for the High and Low Language Facility subgroups. This seems to be largely the result of the three boys in Classes IV and V being in those groups. In the case of the age groups, analysis of variance shows the *difference* in variability to be significant at the .01 level.

Class I, like many other categories near the ceilings of scales, does not discriminate well within itself. While it was relatively easy to place on the scale most of the fathers whose jobs, as lawyer, engineer, etc., were well defined by their titles, it was quite difficult, in the absence of detailed knowledge of the nature of jobs and incomes, to assign some of the boys who were on the borderline between Classes I and II. Perhaps it does not really matter, inasmuch as these two groups in any normally distributed population are often considered together as "Up top." However, some analysis may be of interest to sociologists.

Forty-six of the boys (82 per cent) were already in the "Upper-class" and "Upper-middle-class" ranks, I and II, by 1964–1965, as were the fathers of fifty-one of the fifty-six (91 per cent) in the boys' youth. As contrasted with the fathers' situation, the prevalence among the boys of "middle management" and other positions which are generally assigned to Class II may represent a change in available jobs and/or a trend toward less competitiveness, a different attitude toward the importance of work as a value, or a recognition of a wider variety of occupational satisfactions available in modern life. The boys have tended thus far to spread out a bit more in kinds of occupation than their fathers. Some of the differences in level achieved may be due to normal "regression," i.e., the expectation that sons of high status men will tend to fall back somewhat toward the average of the general population. Many of the differences in occupational level can be accounted for by age differences. For example, while there are none of the boys who are college presidents, deans, or directors of research institutes[1] and only one who is a full professor and university department head, the individual fathers who held these ranks were older than *their* sons are today. The sons, however, are approximately their fathers' equals in education. Time will undoubtedly change the occupational status picture. Even as it is, occupational *choices* are generally consistent with parental social patterns.

---

[1] During manuscript preparation at least one boy in the older group achieved this status.

Occupations of Fathers and Sons

In this professionally oriented group, in which the cultural milieu seems to have played a large part in the educational and occupational histories of the boys, it might be expected that many boys would follow their fathers' occupational choices specifically. This, in fact, turns out to be the exception rather than the rule. Speaking now of the entire group, we find that:

Two boys whose fathers were lawyers are themselves lawyers, partners in their respective firms, but neither in his father's firm.

One boy is a junior officer in the bank of which his father was president.

One boy, like his father, is a university professor of economics, but not in the same university nor the same economic specialty.

One boy is a technical salesman, like his father, but in a different firm.

Two other young college professors have perhaps chosen teaching because of family patterns, but are in different disciplines from their fathers'.

And there the specifics of family patterning seem to end. The rest is apparently a matter of similarity of broadly cultural and intellectual interests, aims, or talents.

The few cases of marked difference between father and son are relatively evenly distributed on the Language Facility Scale.

Life Styles of Two Generations

The culture-patterns of the fathers' generation generally included completion of education, and perhaps establishment in a career, before marriage. Many of the boys, however, were married while in graduate school, or even as undergraduates. Some of their children were born while the boys were still full-time graduate students, a situation very rare in the fathers' generation.

The ages of all the fathers at the time of the boys' grade school years were not available, but the average age was probably a little higher than that of the boys in 1964–1965, with a narrower range and smaller standard deviation. The younger boys were considerably younger when interviewed in 1964–1965 than the fathers were in those boys' elementary school years. Only a few of the oldest boys had children old enough to have completed the school's sixth grade; they and a few others also had children in the school or of grade school age; most had younger children, if any. The moving average of the fathers' ages, of course, would have been that of "men with elementary school children" and would probably have represented a calendar spread different from that of the boys, which had a fifteen year range in birthdates in the single year 1964–1965.

Age, Career Interruptions, and Status Earning Opportunity

Since the forty-six boys who were placed with such accuracy as was possible in *Socioeconomic Classes I and II* turned out, in this restricted section of the occupational spectrum, to present a picture of high correlation of achievement with age group, further examination of this problem promised to be of interest. (The inclusion of the ten boys in Classes III, IV and V made the *over-all* difference very slight.) The distribution as of 1964–1965 is probably a temporary one, in any case, since some of the boys, particularly the younger ones, can be expected to move up a step or two in the occupational scale. Nevertheless, the picture is so striking that it should be noticed.

DETAIL FROM TABLE 19

Occupational Status

Age Group	Class I	Class II	Total
Older Half	16	6	22
Younger Half	8	16	24
Totals	24	22	46

$x^2 - P < .05$, slightly $> .01$.

Service Interruptions of Careers

Service interruptions affected both generations. A few fathers' careers (especially those of fathers of the older group) were interrupted by military or alternate service in connection with World

War I, but the lives of the boys in the younger group were generally affected more than were *their* fathers' lives. In this Philadelphia-based community, several of the boys, members of The Society of Friends (Quakers), or in sympathy with its position, were granted Conscientious Objector status by their draft boards, but many of those so classified spent time in "alternate service," either voluntary or required, about equivalent to the time spent in the Armed Forces by their classmates. Some were not drafted or enlisted in either capacity—five in the older and six in the younger group. From the point of view of this inquiry the two types of interruptions of civilian careers were treated together. (Table 22.)

Table 22

YEARS OF MILITARY OR ALTERNATE SERVICE

Years	Number of boys	Total years
0	11[a]	0
0.5	3	1.5
1	7	7
2	24	48
3	6	18
4	3	12
16 (Army, 1st career)	1	omitted
Unknown	1	omitted
Totals	56	86.5

For 43 boys in noncareer service:
Total man-years   86.5
Mean, in years   2.0

[a] 5 Older group, 6 Younger group.

The number of years since high school graduation (assumed age 18) was calculated for each boy. The number of years interruption of career for military or alternate service was subtracted. A mean of 13.7 years available for *higher education and career achievement* was found for fifty-four subjects. (One was omitted as having had sixteen career years in the Army and one because data on military service was incomplete.) A mean of 16.4 available years was found for the twenty-six (of twenty-eight) older boys while for the twenty-eight younger boys the mean was 10.8 years. With the total mean assigned a value of 100, an index of years available for study and work was calculated for the older and the younger groups, 120 and 79, respectively, the difference being forty-one points (Index A, below, A_1—Older, A_2—Younger).

Similar calculations were made after further deducting the number of years post-high school education for each boy, giving a mean of 8.1 years available for *employment alone* for the group as a whole, 10.6 years for the Older group and 5.9 years for the Younger group. An index calculated on this second basis showed a difference of forty points. (Index B, B_1—Older, B_2—Younger)

$$\text{Index A: Total} = 100, A_1 = 120, A_2 = 79, \text{Diff.} = 41 \text{ points}$$
$$\text{Index B: Total} = 100, B_1 = 113, B_2 = 73, \text{Diff.} = 40 \text{ points}$$

Thus, a relationship between age and socioeconomic class achievement might well be expected.

CHILDHOOD IQ AND ADULT ACCOMPLISHMENT

Contrasts Which Raised Questions

A striking parallel in life histories between the two boys with language rank No's. 12 and 50 threw into bold relief the extreme difference in their childhood IQ's. These boys, not close friends, were about three and a half years apart in age but four classes apart and so not in high school, college or medical school together. They attended the same secondary school which frequently sent its more able students, including these two, to the same small university. There the boys made almost identically outstanding records (Highest Honors, Phi Beta Kappa, Sigma Xi, and other distinctions) in the demanding premedical course. They attended the same medical school but developed different specialized interests. In 1964–1965 both were engaged in research and appeared likely to achieve distinction consistent with their academic records. The older boy had already begun to do this, with over fifty scientific publications and a national award in his field. The younger scientist had done very well as to publications and recognition considering his age and an extra three years spent in post-doctoral study, but had just accepted his first post-degree position when interviewed in 1965.

The startling contrast of 52 IQ points, based on two consistent Binet tests for each boy, could not be ignored. Subject No. 12, with the higher IQ, achieved his school record with less apparent effort than did Subject No. 50, whose extreme childhood dyslexia left him with residuals such as "rather slow reading speed" and continued "very poor spelling" (his own 1965 appraisal). Still, the harder work was by no means compulsively all engrossing. This young man had a breadth of interests and a pattern of personal-social development which seemed consistent with his other areas of superiority.

Admittedly the comparison here was between the "most gifted subject" (by Binet score criterion only—IQ 185) and the "most successfully rehabilitated extreme dyslexic" (by educational achievement criterion only—two doctoral degrees). While such a parallel and contrast was most unlikely to be repeated, it drew attention to the apparent "ceiling" of IQ 135, only once exceeded, in the Low Language Facility group (see Figure 3, Chapter IV)[2] and suggested a comparative study of IQ's in pairs of dyslexics and non-dyslexics matched as closely as was possible as to educational and career histories.

A Study of Matched Pairs

Given the homogeneity of the population, it proved relatively easy to pair each boy of the Low Language Facility group with a "best match" from among the other two groups on the basis of the history and the 1964–1965 status of each boy. Some of these "matches" were exceedingly close and all seemed adequate for the comparative study. The criteria used were:

Age- $\leqslant$ three calendar years difference.
Years of higher education- $\leqslant$ one year difference, except in three
    cases.

---

[2] The writer has occasionally tested other dyslexics whose Binet IQ's exceeded 135. One, a brother of one of the subjects reported here, achieved a score of 179 at age 7 before reading instruction or formal training in arithmetic.

Type and degree of "difficulty" of college and university attended; e.g., Haverford paired with Swarthmore, Harvard with Yale; wherever possible attendance at the same institutions.

Socioeconomic status—generally either the same or minimally different.

Occupational choice—from "identical" to "closely comparable."

No attempt was made to match personality factors.

Since it was necessary to use for pairing only twenty of the thirty-six boys in the High and Medium Language Facility groups, it was possible to find matching subjects without including the five who had been thought of and taught as mildly dyslexic (see Chapter III), the two whose Binet tests were incomplete, the three youngest subjects, the boy with hearing loss, and five others not needed. (See Figure 7.)

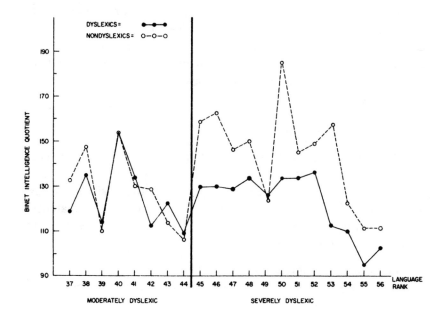

Figure 7. Childhood IQ's of dyslexic boys (Numbers 37–56 on the Language Learning Facility Scale), compared with IQ's of nondyslexic boys (not here identified by number). Subsequent life histories of the paired subjects were closely matched as to age, education, and occupation.

The range of IQ's in the dyslexic group was from 94 to 153, and in the matching group from 111 to 185. In fourteen pairs the IQ differences favored the nondyslexic subjects by from 11 to 52 points, with a median difference of 14.3 points, a mean difference of 22.2 points (t-test—P < .01), and a standard deviation of 12.8 points. In five cases the IQ differences favored the dyslexics by from 2 to 9 points with a mean of 3.6 points (t-test—nonsignificant) and a standard deviation of 3.2 points. In one case only were the IQ's of a pair identical, the pair including the 153 IQ mentioned earlier as the sole score above 135 among the dyslexics. The life histories of these two boys were also strikingly similar.

The t-test shows the difference between the mean favoring the fourteen nondyslexic boys and that favoring the five dyslexic boys to be significant beyond the .001 level.

The relationship of childhood IQ to dyslexia is particularly notice-able in the group of twelve boys rated "severely dyslexic." In only one case, and there by only two points, was the IQ of the non-dyslexic member of a pair below that of the dyslexic. (The "match" in this pair, while rated nondyslexic, was nevertheless a boy who had difficulty expressing his thoughts in words. It is quite possible that he, too, was underrated by the Binet test.) The mean differ-ence favored the nondyslexics by an obviously highly significant 21.9 points. This subgroup is the major source of the difference noted for the Low Language Facility group as a whole (twenty boys), and of the moderate correlation of IQ with language rank previously noted.

Whenever statistical averages are used some loss in significant de-tail is inevitable. A closer look at individuals showed this to be probable in the IQ comparison. In nine of the twenty dyslexic boys' scores the investigator felt fairly secure in judging that the Binet test had, in fact, measured the boys' academic potential adequately. In eleven cases among the dyslexics, however, and at least five among those adjudged nondyslexic, the Binet score had not been an adequate predictor of academic achievement.

For example, there was a difference of 46 points between two "matched" scientists with undergraduate degrees from Swarthmore and Haverford and doctorates from Yale and Harvard. The dyslexic was tested by a very competent outside examiner and the nondyslexic's score was later validated by retest by an outside examiner. Were these two boys as far apart in intellectual ability as their IQ's suggested?

Other differences, both large and small, seemed indicative of the effect of verbal factors on test scores which was not necessarily reflected in ultimate academic achievement. In two cases (Nos. 14 and 22), described in the "Case Notes" in Chapter III, the school may very well have missed opportunities to help two boys with language problems of a dyslexic type. Information suggesting this came to light especially during the follow-up interviews. In another instance, the "match" of the boy with his moderately dyslexic counterpart was particularly close and the IQ figures equally, and very considerably, seemed to have underestimated the potential of both boys of the pair. Binet scores in the low 130's do not lead one to expect distinction in post-doctoral study and research careers such as describe these boys. The examiner (the author in both cases) was certainly unaware of whatever specific "ceiling factor(s)" may have been operating but recalls having been a bit surprised in each instance that the score was not higher for these apparently gifted and creative youngsters.

Two dyslexics made IQ scores below 120 but later earned Ph.D's. from well known universities and achieved professorial rank on university faculties. Had anyone at the school, or any later counselor, discouraged the boys from academic pursuits or advised their parents to do so on the basis of the childhood IQ's, the pressures of "the self-fulfilling prophecy" might have been added to the language burden the boys were already carrying. "College may be too tough for you; graduate school is a most unrealistic idea." Such a statement, or even the attitude behind it, could have discouraged the boys and damaged self-concepts already vulnerable.

A well qualified psychologist would not have used a single IQ figure this way, of course, but might himself have been influenced in his judgment by a boy's performance on such a justifiably highly respected instrument as the Binet, as the school staff may well have been in the case of boy No. 22, for example. Moreover, not all users of test scores are equally sophisticated, nor are most parents in position to thread their ways among the values and limitations of findings or their interpreters, even if scrupulous care is used in not quoting IQ figures. The Binet test is still a much better instrument to use with a language disabled youngster than are classroom group tests, but great caution is always indicated in its interpretation.[3]

PRESENT READING, SPELLING AND PENMANSHIP

The informants reported on the boys' present reading, spelling, and penmanship. These are their subjective judgments; the figures based on them are given for whatever they may indicate (Tables 23 and 24). It is not surprising that significant correlations were found here, and that the relationships of adult reading and adult spelling skills with Language Learning Facility rank are particularly evident. Because of the nature of the distributions, these coefficients of correlation are more suggestive than supportable by the strict canons of statistics.

Table 23

APPRAISAL OF CURRENT READING, 1964–1965

Subject's or Informant's Comments	Number of Boys
Skill and quantity levels high	29
Skill adequate, quantity limited	5
Somewhat hampered by poor skills — slow	14
Very much hampered by skill factors	3
No comment	5
Total	56

Association with language rank
$r = .6846$, $P < .01$

[3] Other intelligence tests, especially the Wechsler instruments in the writer's experience, share some of the Binet's limitations. One should, for instance, be aware of whether the Wechsler Digit Symbol (optional) and Coding subtest scores were included in the Verbal, Performance and Full Scale IQ's, to mention only the two subtests most commonly out of line in dyslexics' score profiles. In the writer's opinion qualitative appraisal from the language learning point of view should always accompany psychometric evaluations, especially those of suspected dyslexics.

Table 24

APPRAISAL OF CURRENT SPELLING, 1964–1965

Subject's or Informant's Comments	Number of Boys
No problem	20
Occasional errors, but readily manageable	11
"Troublesome"	14
"Awful"	5
No comment	6
Total	56

Association with language rank
r = .5493, P < .01.

The dyslexic boys have found many ways of adapting to the difficulties caused by their constitutional make-up. Dan, the lawyer, for example, overcame a speech articulation problem by careful practice. He reported that he took conscious advantage of good instruction in English writing and sought out opportunities for criticism, as on the Law Review in his law school years. He is an avid but not a voluminous reader and does not trust himself to remember large quantities of verbal material as do many of his associates. As a general rule he relies instead, he said, on the rational structure of the law, reasons his way through legal problems, and makes his reading count and his remembering more effective because both are controlled by specific purpose. Not only a successful lawyer and a good "family man," he was also finding time and enthusiasm for many community responsibilities. This is perhaps as good an example as any of the kind of mobilizing force which it seems that many dyslexics learn to use in varied fields of endeavor. The hypothesis that this can be a "serendipitous" effect of the sustained, systematic effort they are called upon to make may at least partly explain the achievements of the young people described here.

FURTHER SOCIOLOGICAL DATA

The boys, and their relatives and friends, supplied a considerable amount of other information about their current statuses, activities, and attitudes. Many informants felt, as did the author, that "just knowing about a person's school history and his job is not enough to give a good picture of him," but practical limitations precluded the making of the kind of "in-depth" studies reported by Roe (1952) or Ginsberg and Herma (1964). Much extremely interesting material came to light in the "open-end" interviews of this study, and much more is available, should circumstances permit its collection and analysis. To round out the sociological picture of the parent-schoolchild era given in Chapter II, some material about the boys' current families is given. No subgroup differences in factors readily measurable, except those related to age, seem to be important or, where tested, statistically significant.

Family Constellations—The Boys as Adults

In 1964–1965 nine boys of varying ages were still bachelors. This made the number of new families forty-seven, nearly the same number as the forty-four families of the parent generation. In 1964–1965 forty of these families had children, with several having a child or two more than did the boys' childhood families. One might guess that when the marriages and child-bearings are complete the school community would have somewhat more than reproduced itself.

Table 25
FAMILY STATUS OF BOYS AS ADULTS, 1964–1965

Marital status	Number of boys
Unmarried[a]	9
Married	44
Divorced, not remarried[a]	2
Divorced, remarried	1
Total	56

[a] At least one married since data collection.

Relationship of the Boys to the School Community

Life has, of course, taken many of the boys to other parts of the country, and one to Canada, to live. As far as could be determined, most of them remembered the school with varying degrees of pleasure, affection, nostalgia and/or enthusiasm, even when, as in some cases, the memory was dim or there was criticism of some aspects

Table 26
NUMBER OF CHILDREN OF 47 BOYS, 1964–1965

Children per family	No. of families
0	7
1	3
2	19
3	12
4	4
5	1
6	1
	47

Mean — 2.2 children
S.D. — 2.5

of the school experience. Several boys living at a distance expressed intense regret that they did not have this school or one like it for their children, although others genuinely preferred a more conventional environment for their youngsters. There were several instances reported of community activity in local schools including school board membership "to try to make them more like Rose Valley," and one boy purposely chose as his home a community in which the public schools are "as much like Rose Valley as possible."

Several boys whose work keeps them in the Philadelphia area have settled within walking or driving distance of the school, and at least one of them chose between a Midwestern and a Philadelphia job on the basis of having the school available. To the considerable number of children in the school each year whose parents spent part of their childhood there, the fifty-six boys of this study have contributed their share. The level of the boys' participation in the affairs of the school parallels that of the parent generation; in 1964–1965 at least five boys' families were represented on the school's Board of Directors; one boy was Chairman, one was Treasurer.

CASE HISTORIES OF FOUR FAMILIES

Longitudinal descriptions of four families, each consisting of three living generations, with the "boys" now the middle generation, provide examples of the human realities behind the statistics, and are historically and sociologically more comprehensive than the case materials scattered through the earlier parts of the report.

Of course, no one of the families in the study population is in every way similar to any other. Those described below were chosen partly for their comparability with one another. The families described are also as representative of the group as could be selected. Each of the other forty families shares many characteristics with them. In the four families two boys were in the High Language Facility group, three in the Medium, and three in the Low group. One boy was an only child, two families had two sons each, and one had three boys. There were no siblings not in the study population. A factor in case selection here, as in the Case Histories of Chapter V, was the probable identification of subjects by readers of the report. Almost all the material here reported is either already known to probable readers from the school community (the ones most likely to recognize the subjects) or is, in a sense, a matter of "public record." The rest, such as discussion of dyslexic patterns in the families and in the boys' childhoods, or residual problems, is material which does not objectionably invade the privacy of the individuals involved. Families were chosen in which both the parents and the boys have long been quite aware of the nature of dyslexia and their relation to the problem. They recognize also the success with which those of the boys who had been seriously affected have come to terms with their difficulties. As one boy said, "I have nothing to be ashamed of." And he added, with a wry smile, "Dyslexia has happened to some of the very best people!" The text which follows has been approved by at least one member of each family.

One family's history, from the older half of the group, was in some ways culturally transitional between the patterns of the parents' and the boys' generations discussed earlier. The father was five years late getting his undergraduate degree, and the mother three years late, in both cases partly because of wartime interruptions (World War I). Each had been one year accelerated in high school. The mother had worked four years after marriage before the elder son was born in 1927. The father achieved his master's degree just before the birth of the second son in 1929, while the mother did not earn hers until the boys were in sixth and fourth grades, respectively. Both parents were closely connected with the school.

The elder son completed the sixth grade at the school, finished high school one year accelerated (nontypical for the school's boys), spent fourteen months of World War II in the Navy, two semesters of it in college, and was still one year accelerated on college graduation. He married at 21 (compared to his father's 26), spent four years earning his Ph.D., and entered his first job with one child already born and two others to follow within three years. In 1964–1965 he was a staff scientist in a nonprofit research organization. He chose his place of residence partly because its public school system had basic features similar to those of The School in Rose Valley.

The younger boy in this first family completed the eighth grade at the school, and with some extra work entered the tenth grade in high school, maintaining this acceleration through college. He, also, was married at 21, and the couple had one child by the time the man had achieved his doctorate and his wife her master's degree, six years later. Another child was born two years later. A conscientious objector, this man had career interruption for neither military nor alternate service. He is an associate professor at his former college, and was in part motivated to accept this position so that his children might attend the school, with which at the time of the study he and his wife were identified in much the same ways as were his parents in his boyhood.

The latter boy seemed to the author mildly dyslexic with some residual spelling difficulties, while his brother, despite early speech problems, had no apparent residual symptoms. There is considerable family history of a variety of language problems. Mild symptoms in the children's generation have responded well to preventive measures of phonetic and linguistic orientations in their respective schools.

A second family from the older group of boys consisted of the father, an engineer with B.S. degree, already established in his profession when his three sons were in the school, the mother, with two years of college, first a secretary and then for many years an unusually expert teacher in the school, and the three boys. Of these the eldest, severely dyslexic, spent two post-high school years in the Navy, secured his bachelor's and master's degrees, and is a doctoral candidate. He taught in junior high school and became a principal in the metropolitan school system, with special interest in culturally and emotionally handicapped children, and was in 1965 a public relations representative of the Superintendent of Schools, continuing to hold his rank as "principal." He also operated the summer day camp of The School in Rose Valley for several years and was in 1964–1965 Chairman of the school's Board of Directors. The second boy in the family, a precocious reader, finished school, college, and medical school with highest honors, served two years as a doctor in the Navy, and is now engaged in medical research, having received during the period of our follow-up study an important national award in his field. He was also a member of the Board of Directors of the school in 1964–1965. The third boy, considered slightly dyslexic by the author, completed college with a major in theater arts before serving two years in the Army and spent several years as a professional actor. In 1964–1965 he had become established very successfully in a "middle management" level job in business. All three boys are married and have children. Of the children in elementary or secondary school, two daughters of the oldest boy and a son of the middle, nondyslexic, boy have had language difficulties severe enough to require special help. There are some other relatives, also, who have apparently had dyslexia-related troubles of one sort or another.

A third family includes a boy at the middle of the age distribution, whose background is strongly academic, with his father a Ph.D. college professor and his mother an M.A. school counselor. This boy, an only child, entered the school in the fourth grade as a very severe dyslexic. The school was chosen for him both because of his special need for its language program and for the total school program which seemed to suit his personal requirements. Highly motivated from early childhood toward excellence in performance and achievement, he overcame his reading problem well before eighth grade "graduation," read omnivorously but with only moderate speed, and continued to have difficulty with spelling. His academic career was very similar to that of the middle brother in the family just described, with similar honors from the same institutions. (These boys are obviously the pair referred to at the beginning of the IQ study, above.) The one boy of the fifty-six who had earned two doctorates, he had, when interviewed, just finished his residency in a well-known hospital and received an appointment as an assistant professor in a university, where he was to combine teaching in medicine with continued research in basic science. He reported that he still read "too slowly," and less than he would like to, and that while he found composing fairly easy he still had extreme difficulty with spelling. By 1965 he was married and had two preschool children. Some language problems of typical but non-disabling sorts have been reported among relatives.

A comparable family (the fourth) from the younger age group consists of the father, an economist, well-established in his field during his boys' school years, the mother, a college graduate who was a part-time staff member at the school, and two sons. The elder, perhaps mildly dyslexic, entered the school in third grade, partly because of a speech problem which was soon overcome, completed its seventh grade, graduated from high school and an academically demanding college, tried engineering in industry, spent two years in the U.S. Coast and Geodetic Survey, and then returned to an early interest in geology. He secured his master's degree in this field, was a college teacher at the instructor level, Class II on the occupational scale, at the time of data collection and analysis but very soon afterward rated Class I, having been awarded his doctor's degree just after the close of the study. With a post-doctoral research fellowship granted for the next year, he was, in a sense, at the beginning of his research career, although he already had had both American and foreign experience in his field. A bachelor at the time of data collection, he was married shortly thereafter. His younger brother, a moderately dyslexic member of the Low Language Learning Facility group in school, though even then with obviously high potential, had by 1965 apparently overcome most of his handicap. He was able to read in three languages other than English (atypical for the dyslexic group), but still had some characteristic problems with English spelling and penmanship. He was graduated, with honors, from the same college as his brother and from medical school. In 1965 he was just completing four years of Army service in medicine and was about to enter his final year of residency, looking forward to specialized research and practice in a university setting. By 1966 he was a candidate for his second doctorate. He was married, and had three children, with a fourth born soon after the study closed. This family provides an example of the changes still going on in the statistical base, which would alter figures somewhat were the study to be supplemented by further follow-up. In this total family, as in the other three, there were some language and laterality problems, mostly of nondisabling kinds or degrees.

ATTITUDES TOWARD "SUCCESS"

To what extent were these fifty-six boys "force fed," or overmotivated toward "success"? In the judgment of the investigator and other school staff members, probably not more than two or three of the boys could have been rated "very competitive" in their personal orientation during their elementary years, although most of them enjoyed minor competitions. With a few exceptions, distributed throughout the Language Facility groups, they were not "top men" in their high school classes; a few received exceptional honors and distinction in college; more began to distinguish themselves in graduate school, others still later; many still play the success theme in low key or seem to disregard it entirely. It was part of the school and parent consensus that good work in any field was important for its own sake; the school gave achievement tests but no "grades." Most of the adults thought that competitive effort should be based on one's own past and directed toward one's ego-ideal, and that good grades in the "next school" would be fine but were not essential, until, perhaps, in late high school or college years.

This general attitude seems to have been internalized by most of the boys. One of them, a quietly successful lawyer, high on the Language Facility Scale, expressed it thus, "One of the most important values which I developed in the school was that one can confidently approach jobs with the assumption that they will be interesting."

It was this sort of attitude which stimulated the boys in the first family described in the preceding section to accelerate in high school; they reported being eager to get on to college and scientific endeavor as soon as possible. Their parents, having experienced early mild acceleration without disaster and later scholastic interruption with profit, reported that they had been "pleased" with their sons' plans, but had given considerable thought to the nonintellectual aspects of the boys' maturity before giving approval for acceleration. They also reported being very happy to see that the boys were willing, even eager, to spend a year or so more than the minimum time on their graduate studies. There was certainly no pressure here, other than the generally high but realistic expectations characteristic of the family's cultural milieu. The family attitude was expressed by the older boy in his 1965 interview (shortly before he was appointed director of a scientific research institution): "I remember learning, both at home and at school, that it's important to do as well as you, yourself, can and not to worry about the other guy. I still believe this."

Chapter V

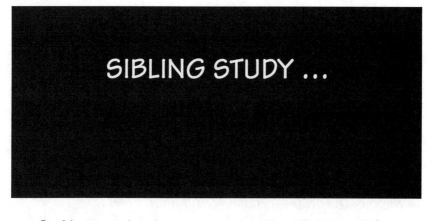

SIBLING STUDY ...

In this population there were ten families which contributed more than one son each to the study. Two families had three sons each, eight had two sons each.

In one of the latter families the boys were not genetically related, one being an adopted son. It was, incidentally, this family which insured caution in the investigator's early interest in the theory of the genetic etiology of language problems. Considering the now apparent high incidence of such problems in the general population it is not at all impossible to conceive that both boys could, by chance alone, have had severe language disabilities of primarily genetic origin, though from entirely different hereditary sources. However, this family is one to which the school and the study owe a considerable debt for many reasons, not least of which was the stimulus they unwittingly provided from the beginning for looking critically at the genetic, emotional, environmental, and educational factors, all of which shaped the boys' lives. They helped to insure the program from the beginning against the temptations of simple answers and panaceas. These brothers, so different in many fundamental ways, also had much in common. The diagnosis of specific language disability was made by two different neuropsychiatrists with several years intervening. The first boy, despite some persisting language problems, achieved his Ph.D. from a famous university and became a faculty member, with professorial rank, in the chemistry department at another university. The other boy graduated from secondary school and became a machinist; he was still in training when interviewed, having made a very good adjustment to life, one which is satisfactory to him and his family. He has the respect and affection of his former schoolmates, as well as of later associates.

One of the surprising findings of this study was the extent of the sibling similarity in the other nine families, that between the pairs of brothers in the two-sibling families being particularly marked, especially in Binet IQ scores. Although the number of families is small, the extent of the similarities seems to warrant mention (Table 27).

Intelligence Quotients—Terman-Merrill Binet, Form L

Of the seven *pairs* of biological brothers tested at different times but by the same examiner, six pairs had IQ's showing one brother differing from the other by less than five points. Within the limits of the test's accuracy, these could be considered to range from identical scores, as in two pairs they literally were, to those with nonsignificant differences. The separate averages of paired scores in the six families ranged from 131 to 159.5 with three pairs in the 130's, one in the 140's and two in the 150's. One member of the seventh pair, where there was large childhood IQ discrepancy between the brothers, was the boy with severe hearing loss and the almost certainly unreliable Binet score referred to earlier. The IQ difference in this pair undoubtedly exaggerated, but to an unknown degree, any true difference which may have existed between these brothers; similarity of their early inherent intellectual power must remain a matter of speculation based on their later histories, which are far less dissimilar than their childhood IQ's.

One *trio* of brothers had scores which showed marked differences —more differences, perhaps, in these scores than in many of their other characteristics. They ranged widely in Language Rank, in the same order as their IQ differences. In the second trio the middle-scoring boy stood three points above one brother and five points below the other. Had either the lowest or highest scoring brother not been a part of the study, there would have been another pair consistent with the six above, a truly astonishing proportion of this small group.

It should be emphasized again that these tests were given at sep-

Table 27
SIBLING STUDY — 22 BOYS, 1964–1965

Family	Son	Age	Language rank	Point difference in IQ	Years of post h.s. education	Highest degree	Boy's occupation	Father's occupation
I	1	38	52		7	MEd	School principal	Engineer
	2	37	12	>5	8	MD	Research Scientist	
	3	35	34		5	BA	"Middle Management"	
II	1	36	37		8	PhD	Full Professor	Business
	2	34	30	8	4	BA	Technical Assistant	
	3	30	31	(see text)	5	BA	Secondary Teacher	
III	1	40	53		8	PhD	Asst. Professor	Lawyer
	2	34	54	1	2	None	Technical Trainee	
IV	1	35	21		8	PhD	Asst. Professor	Lawyer
	2	31	29	>5	5	BA	Government Scientist	
V	1	38	45		7	MBA	"Medium Business"	Assoc. Professor
	2	34	14	0	10	PhD	Asst. Professor	
VI	1	37	11		8	PhD	Research Scientist	Engineer
	2	35	33	3	8	PhD	Assoc. Professor	
VII	1	36	51		5	BS	Personnel Manager	Economist
	2	34	41	0	10	PhD	Research Scientist	
VIII	1	35	48		7	LLB	Lawyer	Lawyer
	2	32	47	4	7	DD[a]	Secondary Teacher	
IX	1	32	6		7	MA	City Planner	Assoc. Professor
	2	26	13	4	3	Undergrad.	Garage, Museum	
X	1	31	32		7	MA[b]	Instructor in University	Economist
	2	29	40	2	8	MD	Physician	

[a] MA ⎫ Additional degrees granted shortly after close of study.
[b] PhD ⎭

107

arated times and that the prevalence of striking sibling similarities came into focus only in connection with the current study, many years later. Such results as these, because of the small numbers involved, must be accepted with appropriate caution, but they cannot fail to be of more than passing interest.

Educational and Vocational Achievement of Siblings

The first trio of brothers has already been described in the family histories as have two of the pairs. One boy from each of two other pairs appears in the five case histories. The accompanying table includes them and the other families.

Sociological Data

The table gives pertinent facts of a "public-record" nature about the sibling groups, omitting, for reasons having to do with confidences and identification, IQ figures and the investigator's judgments as to socioeconomic class status. To point out the interfraternal, as well as the intergenerational similarities shown in the table would be to belabor the obvious. One wonders what the picture of siblings and first cousins among the boys' children will be like twenty-five years hence.

Chapter VI

CONCLUSION...

Summary

This study has documented the unity-in-diversity and, even more, the diversity-in-unity, of a highly homogeneous group of fifty-six young men from 44 families, for the most part white, American, Protestant, professionally oriented, highly educated, intelligent, "intellectual,"[1] upper-middle-class, financially solvent but not wealthy, educationally nonconventional, and individualistic. The report has been concerned with language learning in the young men's educational and occupational histories, under circumstances which began with early study, appraisal and, where indicated, special treatment of language disabilities.

Because of lack of enough exact data and experimentally designed controls, and because of shortage of time and financial resources, no attempt has been made to measure the adequacy of this treatment specifically. However, it has been observed that, for whatever reasons, the boys who were early diagnosed as having severe to moderate specific language disabilities (dyslexia) have achieved at least as high levels of education and socioeconomic status as their more linguistically facile schoolmates. On the other hand, several individuals still find that some of the residuals of their language problems are sources of difficulty in their current lives. They have not been stopped in their careers. Occasionally they have been slowed in their progress and some may even have been stimulated to

---

[1] For distinction between these categories, see Barzun (1959).

greater, more determined, and more systematic effort by the necessity of facing the language problems, of which they have been keenly aware. Their persistence and their parents' support were vital ingredients in their achievements.

It may be that one of the school's most valuable contributions was to the self-concepts of the dyslexic boys, a persistent faith in their intelligence and capacity to achieve, transmitted to the boys directly and indirectly. Important as encouragement was, however, it would probably not have been adequate by itself. It was necessary to work toward eventually transcending their self-doubts by convincing them with demonstrations of their progress toward competence. In Aldous Huxley's words, "It is no good knowing about the taste of strawberries out of a book."[2] Convincing the boys of their progress was not always quick or easy, even when the evidence was clearly before them.

This study gives a clear answer to the originally stated hypothesis that "dyslexic boys of normal or superior intelligence necessarily have poorer prospects for educational and occupational achievement than do nondyslexic boys," and to its elaboration in the null hypothesis form. It can now be said with a high degree of confidence that dyslexic boys *need not* be considered poor risks for academic and occupational pursuits. (It may also be appropriate to repeat that the author and many of her colleagues have seen numerous other cases of proportionately good results among children similar to those studied here and among children with less favorable hereditary and environmental circumstances.) Clinicians working in the field of dyslexia may find justification in this study for more hopeful prognoses. Teachers, as well as parents and their dyslexic children, should derive encouragement from the history of the boys of an earlier generation at the School in Rose Valley.

As a final·illustration the following paragraphs are reprinted from the June, 1966, issue of the *Parents' Bulletin* of The School in Rose Valley, issued on the retirement of Miss Rotzel as principal. They were written by one of the boys in the study.

---

[2] Huxley, J. (ed.) 1965. *Aldous Huxley: 1894–1963*. New York: Harper and Row. (Quoted in review by Richard P. Marsh in *ETC.*, A Review of General Semantics, 24:105–111.)

Grace Rotzel

She was "Rotzy" to the children who first came to The School in Rose Valley 37 years ago. She showed us about growing things and taught us the sword dance, and took us on bird walks. She understood us, and we knew it. Through her vision and enthusiasm a school was created in which learning was exciting and in which boys and girls could "stretch," physically, creatively, and intellectually.

Grace convinced many parents that this was a good place for their children. They built, puttered [that is, maintained the physical plant by organized week-end labor], raised money, ran fairs, and contributed their time and effort in myriad ways—they got involved.

From the very beginning, Grace brought to Rose Valley a very special group of teachers. Men and women who were willing to work for little in the way of monetary reward because they valued children and believed in the school. She encouraged them to read, to discuss, and to try new ideas. She stimulated their thinking and created an atmosphere in which teachers could develop and grow in knowledge and ability.

Thus, she's helped us all—children, teachers, and parents—with a word of encouragement, a question that gets to the heart of things, a smile, or just by listening. She seldom imposes her notions, but rather shares some basic truths and encourages each person to implement these in the way best suited to him.

Just as the school is Grace, so it is also the sum total of all those who have been a part of it. With patience and understanding she has focused the talents of many people on the task of helping children. For this has been her great strength: to utilize the best that each person has to offer. We are all the richer for knowing her.   Jerry ———

June, 1966.

This is an example of the adult writing of one of the boys who have been described. It is, one might say, the latest "composition" by "Jerry," one of the earliest dyslexics in the study. "Jerry" has appeared many times in our narrative—among the severely dyslexic boys, among the successful young men, and as part of Family II in the family histories. He has been close to the school during much of his life and has known Miss Rotzel in the full gamut of capacities: as one of her early students; as a parent of three recent students; as a professional colleague; as Chairman of the Board of

Directors of the school at the time of her retirement (in which capacity, although he would not put it this way, he was, technically, her "employer"). There is no doubt that he knows his subject and that he can write. Perhaps the reader will find here an epitome of the possibilities of adult accomplishment of dyslexic boys.

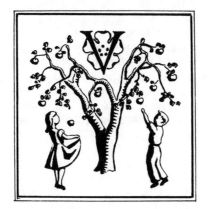

We shall not cease from exploration
And the end of all our exploring
Will be to arrive where we started
And to know the place for the first time.

T. S. Eliot*

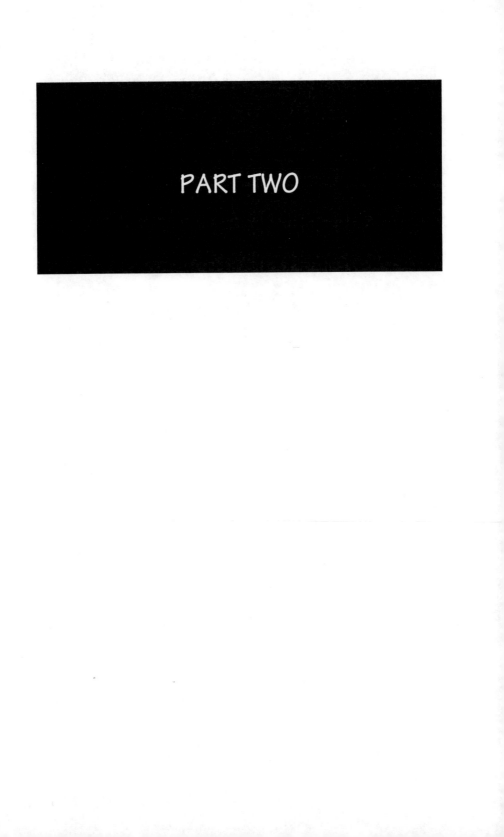

PART TWO

Chapter VII

THE MEN'S FURTHER ACCOMPLISHMENTS BY 1989–1990

INTRODUCTION

The new chapters of this second edition of *Developmental Language Disability: Adult Accomplishments of Dyslexic Boys*, now retitled *Dyslexia over the Lifespan: A Fifty-Five-Year Longitudinal Study*, will bring to a close the report of a longitudinal account spanning 55 years of the lives of its subjects, together with reflections on the connections of that history with the field of dyslexia. There will be a summary of the changes that have occurred in the group of 56 men in the 25 years since they were reported upon so intensively in 1968. The resurveyed group was comprised of 44 respondents in 1990. These groups will be referred to as n56 and n44, respectively, with the latter group providing the new material for the forthcoming chapters. There will be a summary indication as to what has become of the twelve men no longer under scrutiny. Furthermore, since this is truly a continued story, a recent reading of Part I will make the cross-references in the case material more meaningful.

This new edition's added chapters will first give readers information through 1990 on the well-being and whereabouts of the members of the 1965 group, a summary of their educational and vocational achievements in the past quarter-century for comparative references, and, to round out the sociological aspect of that picture, some account of their personal and social interests. We will also consider replacement on the Language Learning Facility Scale. This unique scale was devised in 1965 specifically for this study, as described in Chapter 3, page 34. It provided, within the limits of the available data in 1965, a composite measure of the ease or difficulty with which each subject, as a child, had acquired the skills needed in the use of his first language, relating his position to the other subjects and to the field of dyslexia. In the current investigation each man is still frequently identified by symbol with his original high, medium, or low scale status (LLF I, II, or III) so that one can readily keep in mind the particular relationship between some aspect of his present and his own linguistic past in this story as a parallel undercurrent, a critical dimension which might otherwise be undervalued.

We will also consider what the further life history of the group of subjects discussed in Rawson 1968 tells about the validity of assessment in dyslexia, especially with respect to academic and vocational potentials. Finally the relationship of the study to the entire field of dyslexia including the newer findings in the scientific disciplines related to the language function will be explored.

SOURCES OF INFORMATION

We can now use a longer historical review that takes in all, or a large part of, the working life of each man and of the investigator. In addition to the extra 25 years of data, the perspectives of time have made possible a richer and more complete view of both the accomplishments and the quality of life of the men at full maturity. There are marked changes to examine in the larger culture, but especially developments in the theoretical and practical understanding of language learning from the days of Orton to the present. However firmly based in fact, today's qualitative judgments must still be partly subjective, and so every effort must be made for them to be consistent with the evidence shown in our enlarged population of knowledge and experience. In the 1990 report, the qualitative judgments have become paramount, and so this is properly a descriptive, not a statistically analytic, presentation.

Because in the late 1980's the original investigator was still in active practice as a writer and researcher, she felt some responsibility for rounding out this part of her interests. Of those who urged that the 1990 follow-up study be undertaken, one of the group, a scientist, was particularly persuasive. Severely dyslexic as a child, included in Language Learning Facility Group III and now a research physician, the man called Ralph had taken a special interest in this project from the beginning.

In 1986, at The School in Rose Valley (SRV), Ruth Goodenough had conducted a survey (Appendix A) of the former students of the school. As a member of the school staff Ms. Goodenough was made aware of our follow-up study, and she shared those alumni responses that were pertinent to our study. The responses gave additional information that enriched our knowledge of the past years. The particulars of her survey often filled in the open-ended and unasked questions of our own 1990 questionnaire. Edith Klausner, the school's principal, was also helpful in the use of the school's records.

In 1989, the author wrote to the original subjects asking for a postcard reply as to whether they would be interested in participating in an update of the study. The response was gratifyingly large and enthusiastic, and so a questionnaire requesting information concerning their educational achievements, occupational and professional activities, special honors, marital, and family status was developed and refined (Appendix A). Several open-ended questions were included to elicit responses on the quality of their lives, their interests and enthusiasms at this stage of their careers, and their thoughts on their facility in language functioning. The written responses to the questionnaire and other inquiries were full of personal detail. Also included in their contributions to the project were telephone calls and spontaneous personal interviews.

All names are fictitious, except for "Jerry" who is so often mentioned in Part I, and Peter Olmsted, to whom the book is dedicated. The pseudonyms remind everyone of the realness of the people behind the statistics. Names are useful in cross-referencing as one reads about the same individuals in occupations, family life, and lifespan effects of dyslexia. To use a name for each of the men on each occasion is not necessary. Vignettes are primarily illustrative of the points to be made in the study based on the extensive case histories collected by the author during a lifetime of observation and friendship with these men. They are also part of the sociological view of this socioeconomic segment of the population so often neglected in research (Introduction, p. xxii). In all instances, confidentiality has been respected to protect the privacy of the subjects.

The kind of holistic education at The School in Rose Valley into which language education was integrated was important for this group of men. However, the success of the language identification and treatment here described was not dependent on the School's curricular background or environmental circumstance, important as these were to each person. In the author's experience, the structured, multisensory approach used in language teaching was found to work anywhere. In her other school and private practice she has worked similarly with people of lower recorded intelligence than most of this particular group of students. The approach has also worked in school settings where personal backgrounds were generally less favorable, and the educators' attitudes less cooperative and even antagonistic.

POPULATION

Of the original 56 men, eight had died before 1990 at ages 37 to 61. Of the remaining 48, four could not be located. The author was in direct contact with 39 men; reliable sources—close family and friends—provided information regarding another five. Given the information provided by the subjects themselves or by others, we still have in the 1990 review, inclusive information (current or as of date of death) for 52 of the original 56 subjects after 55 years.

The 44 men about whom we can now report directly live in the following sixteen states: twelve in Pennsylvania, five in California, five in Maryland, three in New York, two men each in Colorado, Florida, Ohio, Virginia, and Washington, and one man each in Connecticut, Indiana, Maine, Massachusetts, New Jersey, North Carolina, Oregon, and the District of Columbia. In addition, one man lives in New Zealand. Their occupations have also taken many of the men to a number of countries at different times for varying periods. The School's 60th Anniversary Celebration (1989) brought fourteen men from Washington, California, Florida, Maine, and intermediate points.

Of the original Language Learning Facility subgroups (see page 42), there now remain 14 in the "high" group, 13 in the "medium" group, and 17 in the "low" group, the latter being the ones defined in 1965 as "dyslexic." This ranking system had given form for the 1965 statistical analysis which answered the research hypothesis. It must be kept in mind that these subgroupings were established on the basis of information then available.

VALIDITY OF DIAGNOSES

Hindsight would allow us to move Mark [1] and several others in rank order, but these would have been minor statistical adjustments that would have largely offset each other. In personal references the original ranking is used in the progress report chapters as it was in the earlier chapters, making identification less confusing. Later we show a post hoc regrouping.

Had the opportunity permitted the same level of detailed case analysis with the nondyslexic comparison group in 1965 as was done with the dyslexics, an error would have come to light. A false-negative (an instance of a dyslexic who was categorized as a nondyslexic) could have been avoided. Mark [1] attended The School in Rose Valley only through third grade. Mark's Binet Intelligence test score, while somewhat above average at age seven, was marked "an underestimate." (Had he stayed in the school, further testing could have identified him as being dyslexic.) His academic progress was poor, but it was noted in the school records that "emotional problems stop[ped] his learning!" The principal and parents agreed that both Mark and his younger brother, Rob, not included in the study but already in our tutorial group in second grade, might do better in a more formal setting and, as far as we heard, they did. Both boys now hold doctorates of philosophy—Rob's in botany and Mark's in nuclear engineering—and are university department heads. We had thought of the possibility of dyslexia with both, but the emotional problems seemed paramount. It seemed most important to avoid overdiagnosing language learning disability and to obtain the most accurate and unbiased diagnosis possible for each individual. The children at The School in Rose Valley were accustomed to individual teaching or attention for whatever special interests and needs they might have had, not just problem areas. It was the school policy to give help in the language-learning frame of reference whenever needed and possible, whatever the student's other trait-patterns. However, we tried scrupulously to avoid "false positives" in determining a student to be "dyslexic." It may not shake the earth, but it gives Mark interest and the author satisfaction to set straight the "false negative" nearly five decades later.

Mark supplied the missing puzzle piece in 1990, when he said, "I know I'm one of your dyslexics! For three years after we left The School in Rose Valley we [my brother and I] went after school for tutoring to Helen Hall. She worked our very tails off!" Regardless of this extra tutoring, the author, like the elder relative who was the 1965 informant, thought that doing "OK in public schools," graduating from Swarthmore College, and achieving two advanced degrees added up to "no academic problem" for Mark. Dr. Hall and I had long been in close accord in thinking and in using almost identical methods, but we were not in clinical practice together so we were unaware of the identity of each other's individual clients. If we had consulted about Mark specifically, we would have agreed that dyslexia was his basic problem and, as is common, the emotional factors were the result rather than the cause. With a phonological, multisensory approach almost identical to the one at The School in Rose Valley, Dr. Hall had continued the work we had barely started with both boys. It was an old story to her in 1990, at age 98, when we told Dr. Hall what two more of her boys had done. She was glad, but not surprised, to hear of Mark's position in physics and engineering and Rob's in botany. Mark, now holding a doctorate in philosophy, Department Head of Nuclear Engineering, recipient of Sigma Xi, Tau Beta Pi, and The Lloyd Carter Award, and an Atomic Energy Commission Fellow in 1990 said, "I still have some difficulty reading. Sometimes I swap the order of the letters and so misread the words. I am still a 'slow' reader and have trouble spelling, so I always use the spell-checker on my computer." These are typical comments expressing the pervasive and continuing effects of diagnosed childhood dyslexia, a topic which recurs throughout the text.

ADDITIONAL EDUCATIONAL ACHIEVEMENT

Once the students were ranked using the original scale in the 1965 study, educational achievement was analyzed in detail, and so this seemed to merit first follow-up attention in 1990. The actual number of "years worth" of credits reported by 1990 was spread so evenly among the men in the Language Learning Facility Groups that refiguring all the groups' averages made little difference in the relative standing of the group. That difference did, however, accentuate the increase in Group III's lead from 6.0 as their average number of years of graduate school to 6.35 "years worth" in the rating index.

During the past quarter-century, after professional level academic status had been achieved by our subjects, further study was often mentioned or implied, but with the men for whom academic considerations were appropriate, amassing of "credit-hours" had become less relevant. A few of the 44 men in the 1990 study required additional degrees for specific purposes. One man, who already had his medical degree, earned another doctorate in philosophy; another secured a doctorate in education; four other men earned master's degrees. All these degrees enhanced their qualifications for teaching. Two of these men were from Group I, one was from Group II, and the remaining three were classified as Group III. Other men reported course work which did not lead to degrees. In addition, one man from LLF II in the original 56, who had died by the time of this update, had finally completed work for his undergraduate degree.

THE EDUCATORS

Many people have asked whether the men in this study chose employment in fields particularly related to problems they had encountered in their childhood. The answer is not a clear-cut no, for special learning needs of students have influenced the job choices and manner of teaching of those engaged in that occupation. None of the men, however, has specialized in the basic instruction or tutoring of dyslexic students, although several of their wives and children are reported to be working as language specialists. Here as elsewhere in their occupational choices, the men's preferences have been determined by their interests which have been neither dictated nor restricted by their being dyslexic. Several have elected primary or secondary education and serve as teachers or administrators. Their responses to recent inquiry show, in general, the kind of informed opinion and attitude toward individual differences in learning that one might expect given their personal experience. In brief, their experience of childhood dyslexia has not propelled any of our subjects into this specialized area of the profession, but does influence the tenor of their occupational lives as educators.

The teaching experience of one man was particularly relevant to this question. The now retired suburban high school principal gained special insight through his very first teaching job at an inner-city school for children with special needs. This is Jerry [III] who was mentioned so often in the 1968 account. Over the next 21 years in the city school system he advanced to being a secondary school principal and finally became the assistant director of public information for the system. He then made what he considered a major career change, moving to a suburban school. The next eighteen years saw him functioning as a junior high school principal and dean of students with eventual retirement at the rank of high school principal. During this latter period he added up his accumulated credits, finished his dissertation, and completed the requirements for his doctorate in education. "I just decided," he said, "to round things out before I retired." As he comments on his continued awareness of his characteristics as a dyslexic, he says, "I have great empathy with the learning disabled students."

Eric, [III] with a master's degree from divinity school, began his teaching career in religious education. After he earned an additional Masters in Education degree, he served for ten years as headmaster of an independent preparatory boarding school. His next appointment, which he still holds, was to the position of headmaster of a complete (K–12) independent school in a large eastern city.

Quite different, but in some sense "grown in the same garden," is Adam [III] who found his B.A. in English literature to be the only degree he needed. During this past quarter-century he has been teaching English in a New England preparatory boarding school where he has ample scope for sharing his varied extracurricular enthusiasms with students.

Martin, [II] returned ten years after his graduation from college to obtain his Masters in Psychology and Guidance degree. He spent 28 years in public schools teaching junior high school social studies. Now retired, he works in professional photography.

SOCIOECONOMIC CONSIDERATIONS

The culture has so changed that in this follow-up report it seems inappropriate to think in terms of socioeconomic categories, as in the earlier study. Here we consider more specific interests and competencies. More occupations than individuals are now listed, for the several, often concurrent, occupations of some men indicate second and third careers. A most striking example of this is the rural farmer-writer-teacher-editor-publisher, Will [I]. The varied occupations, taken together, are the way he creatively makes his living. In each of his undertakings he aims toward professional expertise. For example, he returned to graduate school for a master's degree in education in order to accredit him to direct and teach part-time in a "Rose Valley-type" school, which he helped establish in the interest of his own children and grandchildren. In which single vocational category could he possibly be placed? The occupational versatility of this man would not seem atypical to any former student of The School in Rose Valley.

Also among the secondary school teachers, Patrick [III] was almost as versatile as Will. Essentially, he followed two parallel careers. Beginning as an electronics engineer, he worked in radio for several large corporations. He broadcast news and classical music, wrote and edited a magazine for radio enthusiasts, and established an incorporated club for amateur radio buffs. Facilitated by his 1968 Masters in Education degree, the parallel career in teaching of technologies culminated in a position as a high school industrial arts teacher. Now retired, Patrick uses this background experience to do volunteer boys' club work and intensive counseling. He explained early retirement as resulting from the city schools' "overcrowded . . . mainstreaming" conditions which were too unsatisfactory to bear. He summed up his experience thus, "I have used education as a device for helping young people in many ways. The results give me the greatest satisfaction."

THE PROFESSORS

As with most of the 1990 respondents, so it is among the twelve men of the university-oriented group. Their interest in the SRV study's specific language focus was expressed in personal communication but did not necessarily influence vocational choice. The nature of their varied interests, however, has led them into the academic world where they are, or have been, engaged in research and teaching at professorial levels. From the study's point of view, it is interesting to note that they represent equally (four each) its three LLF groups. Their positions in these groups is unrelated to the effectiveness of their professional accomplishments.

Four of the twelve in this contingent had become medical doctors by the close of the 1965 report period. Each was, in 1990, a practicing physician, a clinical professor in a university medical school, and a researcher in his own specialty. Two of them chose to do intensive post-doctoral study leading to an advanced academic degree. Ralph [III] had already achieved his Ph.D. in biochemistry before 1965, while Dave (pages 48–9) acquired his doctorate with a concentration in pathology in 1967, early in this current report period. The other two men elected to specialize through individual study and clinical experience. Harvey [I] and Sherman [III] have gone on to achieve distinction in pathology and rheumatology, respectively. Readers interested in case history detail can identify in Part I not only Dave, as indicated, but Ralph, Harvey, and Sherman, who appeared anonymously in three of Chapter 4's "Case Histories of Four Families," pages 98–103.

The other university men represent a wide variety of specialized fields. A man of letters [II] teaches language and literature and has contributed many books and papers with literary quality, creativity, and scholarship.

Another man [I] began as an ornithologist, moved briefly into arctic exploration and research, then turned to anthropology where he is now an authority on the cultures, movements, and problems of peoples of river basin societies in Africa. An economist [II] specializes in the economics of east Asia with particular expertise in Korean affairs. The sociologist [III] in the sample researches, writes, and teaches about family and housing problems of city populations in the United States. Mark, the professor of nuclear engineering, is an internationally respected consultant in the field. The group's geologist, Duncan [II], was a professor in a university classroom, but serves now as curator and researcher in a scientific institution where he informs the public about the volcanoes of the world through exhibits, lectures, articles, and books. In this group is Herbert [III] who devotes all of his time to research. He says, "I am doing research on the nervous system of a tiny parasitic worm, using an electron microscope and computers."

The texture of university life apparent in this group is reflected in the questionnaire responses and accompanying resumes and reprints for all twelve men. Here we could list honors, awards, election to learned and scientific societies, fellowships and visiting professorships, consultancies, service on boards and governmental and private commissions, worldwide recognition of expertise, lectures, and speaking engagements. All of these have been reported—some by several respondents. Publications lists some short, some very long, of books, papers, journal articles, reports, and other works of scholarship and personal interest reflect the individuality and diversity we have described. Such achievements, particularly apparent in the academic world, are reported by other men in their occupational areas as well.

A former member of this professorial group is Sid [II] who in many characteristics and interests is still so much a part of the group that he is included with the other twelve. Sid is representative of those who have made major career changes. At age 48, after teaching college biology for 21 years, he had become a tenured full professor. Sid then decided to spend the rest of his working years pursuing his other lifetime interest. A one-man firm, he describes himself as "general carpenter, solving the problems of older houses." In practice this involves using all the skills ordinarily required and supervised by a general contractor. In addition to providing handyman services, he also oversees, or works on, substantial home improvement projects from architectural design to completion. Consultation on the restoration of a university science building involved some engineering knowledge and skill. Meeting the varied challenges of his present occupation, he says, brings him even greater satisfaction than did his earlier laboratory and field research projects. He has simply switched the roles of his vocational and avocational interests. That Sid's wife, also a biologist, is the director of the department in which he formerly taught, adds to the wholeness of the couple's college town life.

Sid's change is reminiscent of Henry's move reported at the end of the 1965 data (Part I, pages 51–52). Henry [III] turned from an active, promising career as a writer and in-house editor of a public relations firm in New York City to establishing a horticultural business that reflected his lifelong interest in gardens and plant life. This business, begun with his wife as a partner, has grown and flourished. His sons have even become second generation partners.

Are such career changes unique or part of a larger pattern? Several possible reasons which both enable and encourage freedom of choices may be evident here: changes in knowledge and in technology, advances in science and medicine, increased general longevity, longer active working lifetime, and relative political and economic stability in our country.

THE SCIENTISTS AND ENGINEERS

Pragmatism, applied scientific research, and engineering seem associated with one another. In our data this orientation is represented by two men from Language Learning Facility Group I and three from Group III who seem to belong together. An independent petroleum geologist, Everett [I], searches out sources of oil and gas especially in the Rocky Mountain area where he loves to live. He bridges the gap between the scientific researchers and the engineers. Roger [III] an engineer, who changed direction at age 54, went from ownership of a light rail line and then a small airport to a consultancy with private clients in an established urban firm, his current place of employment. Railroads have continued to be a central interest. Currently he is working with partners in the planning of rail networking for several eastern cities as well as urban renewal projects in a northern New Jersey city. Using his computer he is able to live and spend much of his time at his home in the Adirondack Mountains.

It was in character for Luke [III], a hydrologist with significant responsibility for the water supply of a large city, to take a year of additional graduate study in hydrology largely for his own information. The credits earned completed the course requirements for his doctoral degree which, however, he had decided not to pursue. Why should he? To prepare a dissertation would be a digression, for his published papers and reports had already demonstrated his ability to produce work of this caliber. Moreover, he was convinced by experience that meeting the doctorate's "dread foreign language requirements" promised more agony than satisfaction. Other things in his life were of more importance.

Chan [I] whose college preparation was as a "physician's assistant" wrote, "Someday I'm going to put all the parts together and make a career out of it." It looks as though he has already done so as a technologist-businessman. As instrumentation specialist at the university where he designs instruments and apparatus needed by medical researchers, he appears to have accomplished his goal. As owner and sole employee of his own company, Chan designs, develops, patents, manufactures, and distributes prototype instruments and their successors.

Stanley [III] retired to sailing and other compelling interests in 1990 after 36 years as an engineer and personnel manager in a large manufacturing corporation. From early childhood, he was clearly in the lower half of the SRV dyslexic group. Stanley obviously uses language well—this was not his problem—rather he had difficulty decoding and encoding language in graphic form. His gift for verbal expression is shown in his recent well-written account of cruising that came with this personal note: "Whatever dyslexia I have, I can tell North from South." This is just as well, for he cruises the whole North Atlantic coast with various friends.

THE LAWYERS

We have four lawyers in this class: two from Group I, one from Group II, and one from Group III. Similar to the professors' course, the route in a lawyer's career after college graduation requires first a law school degree (or degrees) and then the passing of the bar examination. Next comes an opening position in an established law firm, followed by junior, then senior partnership, with some kind of specialization dictated by circumstances and interests. Our four lawyers, each associated with an established firm, followed this path. Promotion to partnership came early to each of them, and each stayed for many years with the firm of his first association.

Russell [I], the first of these men to start practicing, was also the first to

retire "to go sailing" after 36 years of commuting to and from Philadelphia on weekdays. At 60, in 1985, with their children through secondary
school (SRV) and college and established in their own lives, he and his
wife felt free to move to his boat's home port on the eastern shore of
Maryland. In the same spirit as before (Part I, page 103) Russell has said
hard work can be fun if it is interesting, and he still expects each new
experience to be challenging. Wallace [I], after 33 years with one firm,
changed firms in 1988 and, with 35 years of active practice, still shows no
signs of diminishing zest for his legal and community responsibilities.
The third man, Ben [II], is still a partner in his original firm and is head of
its real estate department.

The account of the fourth man, Dan [III], is the sequel to his story
begun in the 1965 study, by which time he had already become a junior
partner in his law firm. As the firm grew, he also grew to become an executive manager in the partnership. Dan had become a specialist in corporate law and securities. At this point, age 48 and after 21 years in law, he
resigned to go into business. Perhaps this mid-course change was analogous to those of Henry, Sid, Roger, and some others. For the next six
years he was president of a company which developed and manufactured
medical specialty devices. At first an independent business, it developed
into a prosperous company with multinational subsidiaries in Canada,
Japan, and Europe and, while under his presidency, merged with a giant
corporation. Dan's next move was to his present less time-consuming,
more flexible program as a financial counselor. He says he is particularly
happy to be free to spend much of his time and energy as a volunteer
consultant for educational and church institutions, principally in financial
and management affairs. "This combines my past corporate legal experience and experience as a businessman. I value the independence and flexibility which this schedule permits me."

PUBLIC SERVICE

Occupationally the remaining subjects of this study, still from all the
groups, show diverse achievements. A city planner [I] in a southern me-
tropolis is an administrator and developer for the area's transportation
systems and their facilities. In the private sector, as an executive director
in a public health agency, one man [II], with local and state responsibilities also reports national affiliations. He has spent some 40 years on the

important problem of lung disease and has seen the spectacular advancement in the understanding and control of tuberculosis as well as the recognition of the problems of lung cancer and other respiratory ailments.

Three men are employed in federal service. One [III] is a management analyst; another [II] has long been concerned with regulation of weights and measures, and the third [II] is an enforcement officer for the Food and Drug Administration.

THE BUSINESSMEN

Others make their living in business. Some work for themselves or in small firms and some in corporate enterprises of varying sizes. There is an owner of a marine store [I], a real estate salesman [I], and a couple of self-employed accountants [II, II]. After some years in sales, one man [I] moved to executive recruitment.

Then there is Jasper [II] who years ago abandoned a stage career to make a living wage. He did better than that in business, eventually becoming an export manager. Now that his two children have their undergraduate degrees, he can spend as much time as he chooses in community theater. Another businessman [II] is an independent computer customer service manager.

CHESTER

A good person with whom to end the tale of what we called in 1965 "adult accomplishments" is Chester [III] for his is a story of still growing success. Perhaps the least "bookish" of the very dyslexic students, he was still "a skilled workman in training" in 1965. He moved on to "work on plant maintenance" where he was reported by a SRV schoolmate to be universally liked and respected. Then came his very significant promotion to be head of the shipping and receiving department of a manufacturing company. He says, "I am still dyslexic, but find that with the computer, the more I work with figures and words the better I get with both." He lists his "greatest satisfactions" thus: "Happy marriage of over 33 years and raising two well-adjusted and happy children." And, obviously, he enjoys having a responsible job that he can do well. Chester reports also that he "enjoys reading as well as making things." Here is life on the upswing for him at age 57.

THE MISSING

This brings to a conclusion the section of our 1990 educational and occupational data collected from 44 active respondents who were in the 1965 study. Unfortunately, we could not ascertain reliable information about the remaining four.

THE DECEDENTS

It will be recalled that Peter Olmsted [III], to whom the book is dedicated, had died before the 1965 report. He was 37 and had achieved his Ph.D. and the university rank of assistant professor of chemistry. The verified educational and occupational information is presented for the remaining seven who have died in the past quarter-century. One of the youngest among these deceased men [II] had finished his undergraduate work (the only additional degree among these seven) and was employed as a lifeguard. One multifaceted young sales executive [II] was an elected member of a suburban school board and had helped to establish inner city youth-centered community and educational projects. There were two engineers: one [I] was employed as a chemical engineer, the other, a physicist/electrical engineer [I], was a self-employed consultant in manufacturing, physics, and engineering endeavors. Two men, both bachelors, were artists: one [I] was a painter and designer; the other [I] was a man who chose to work just enough on casual jobs to be able to follow his personal interests in art, drama, and writing. The seventh man, a professional actor [III], had a significant career as a writer, television and stage actor, and theatrical producer. These lives, too soon ended, had been generally consistent with those of the 44 1990 respondents, and so did not substantially change the whole study's findings.

SUMMARY

For comparison with the statistics in Rawson 1968, the case material we have given includes primarily information updating the figures for those parts of the previous analysis that are relevant in 1990 to the hypothesis—tested and found to be false—concerning "success as the world sees it." (See pages xxiii, 82, 110.) Not only were the conclusions left intact but rather they were reinforced by the updated data. In brief review, six additional academic degrees were reported among the 1990 respondents, with also some years of nondegree study, and one degree earned by a subject prior to his death. Vocational achievement was, by the 1965 socioeconomic numerical classification measurement criteria, now largely irrelevant and out-of-date. Whatever their childhood language-learning facility rating, as society defines career success, individual achievements show the members of the entire group fully comparable with one another in 1990. The casual observer would be unlikely to notice the differences in individual language functioning, which a more astute observer might recognize and which the men, themselves, take for granted. "Of course, not all dyslexics are good academic and occupational risks, but the evidence clearly shows that dyslexics cannot be judged to be poor risks on the basis of language disability alone" (Rawson, 1968, page 82). Thus, the major statistical conclusions of the previous study seem not only validated but strengthened by the further quarter-century of life experience. We will have more to say about this in the next few chapters.

Chapter VIII

QUALITY OF LIFE: FAMILIES, AVOCATIONS, INTERESTS

SOCIOLOGICAL FOLLOW-UP

The study's recently collected material has much more to say about the accomplishments of its men, not so much in statistical as in human terms. I can now talk of representative aspects of their experiences well into maturity, their personal enthusiasms, residual problems, joys and difficulties, and the extent to which dyslexia has affected them. The memories conjured up and the ideas generated by open-ended questions may be difficult to tally and to analyze objectively, but they have the kind of reality about them that gives added dimensionality to the case-history type of evidence. Case history material inevitably involves subjectivity: the informant's, the reporter's, and the reader's. It has a truth of its own which may add to an understanding that goes beyond bare-fact information. In Part II we have been presenting the information in narrative form, but briefly enough for ready comparison with analogous numerical data in Part I.

Such brevity has necessitated omission of the rounded detail needed to show the full sweep of life and activity as it came to the author from these subjects' accounts of their worlds. Ideally, one should meet their wives, children and grandchildren, and their fellow citizens in the communities of which they are part. A sharing of a small portion of the full and generous descriptions of each man's questionnaire and interview responses can describe a few representative parts of their life outside their classrooms and work places and indicate, where appropriate, their ongoing associations with the phenomena of dyslexia. The narrative, even limited primarily to their responses, can give us a sense of these people as the multifaceted and multidimensional human beings they are. In the general quality of their lives these men have had similar experiences. There have, of course, been sorrows, tragedies, difficulties, and stressful times. We have learned not only of their successful and happy experiences but of illness and death of spouses and children, crises accompanying the aging of parents, and discouraging, though fortunately not prolonged, periods of unemployment. Life has not always been rosy, for such is the common lot of mankind. However, the general tone of their lives seems optimistic, full of zest and the satisfactions of family, community, and personal enjoyment.

The reader of this report may be interested to know that of the study's original 56 men, 50 are or have been married while six remained bachelors. Ten men have been divorced, some more than once. Unfortunately now, two men have reported widowhood. Of the twelve men divorced or widowed, six have not remarried. The total number of children of the 56 men is 138, an average of 2.5, which is just about the same size as their families when they were growing up (see page 26). The latest reported count of grandchildren was 47, and as the phrase has it, "still counting." Our group, thus, follows the general family size patterns of their socioeconomic status.

As the families chose where to live, several settled in, or returned to, an area near Rose Valley, so that their children could attend their fathers' former school. In at least one family the school was the deciding factor in choosing between two otherwise almost equally attractive job opportunities. Other families sought out communities with similar "alternative" schools or in a few cases, like Will's, they helped to found or operate such schools themselves. In the study's responses and in the alumni questionnaire many of the men commented upon how much their whole school experience had meant to them.

Two of the adults known particularly by all of our respondents were referred to again and again as important ongoing influences in our subjects' memories. One of these was Grace Rotzel, the principal, and the other was Edward Rawson (the author's father-in-law), himself a retired headmaster, simply called "Mister" by everyone in the otherwise first-name SRV world. The respondents mentioned instances of Grace Rotzel putting her philosophy into daily practice. The availability of "Mister's" wisdom and influence with teachers, parents, and students extended far beyond his shop classes and was specifically recalled by numerous respondents to both questionnaires. It was not only the individualized educational program (including the language tutoring), but the quality of the teaching and interaction of the school family which accounted for many of the warm, varied, and vividly recurring memories of the men's school experiences. Among the alumni, Harvey, an enthusiastic educator himself, had by 1990 become a well-known scientist, a medical school professor, and department head, and was once again the chairman of the SRV's Board of Directors. He gave as a major objective in his life: "Trying to remake the US educational system—at all levels—in the image of SRV!"

FAMILY PATTERNS

Changes in family patterns is another continuing influence on the quality of life and the men's present attitude and actions toward life and living. In their childhood families most of the mothers were primarily homemakers, though several had part-time teaching jobs. Very few had full-time careers outside of the home. In contrast, in this study's generation it is common for both spouses to have equally respected jobs or professions outside their homes. In at least two families both partners work in the same field of interest: one couple as researchers on the same science project, and the other as teachers in the same school department. Sometimes the jobs complement each other in interest, as in Sid's family, or in the practical affairs of running a business as in Henry's household, where the children have also become part of the enterprise.

As the culture continues to change, almost all of our subjects' adult daughters and sons have independent occupations. Several wives and daughters specialize in the teaching of reading or in serving children with special needs, which must strike a responsive chord with our men. The subjects' children's occupations are of a wider variety than those of their parents and more like those of the general population, but, real and fortuitous as SRV school life was, it bears repeating that this study's validity and importance in the field of dyslexia do not depend on its happy surrounding circumstances.

COMMUNITY SERVICE AND AVOCATIONS

Among our subjects, community or other volunteer work is often felt to be so important that it is given the effort and attention of a professional caliber. Though it is frequently undertaken for sheer recreation and enjoyment, very often both kinds of satisfaction are interwoven. The balancing of the quality of life is apparent in the avocational interests of the present group, again, as in Chapter 7, with the dyslexics being publicly indistinguishable from the rest of the peer groups. The men may not deliberately separate their hours into professional, personal, and family time but many find varied satisfaction in responsible activity in the public interest. The wide scope of these interests includes such diverse concerns as public health, citizen action and participation, child care and education, youth groups, and ecological conservation and preservation. Two men, in particular, spoke of their substantial commitment to the development of quality eldercare which shows their appreciation and respect for the individual person and his or her preferred lifestyle.

Conservation is a field of intense involvement for some, but when Everett or Sherman help clear wilderness trails with friends, their reason for spending the weekend on that particular task may well be "just for the fun of it." Campfire cookery or "rehashing the sailing race on the dock" can have a pleasantly mixed flavor of cooperation and competition.

Sailing does seem to be a compelling interest to many of our subjects, from the eulexic sailor Russell to several of the most dyslexic, like Ray, Ralph, and Stanley. Stanley, a bachelor already quoted in Chapter 7, is using his retirement freedom happily. Of his cultural, musical, and outdoor activities his top priority is sailing. Stan writes that sailing through New York Harbor at the helm of one's yacht is a thrill to be long remembered. This yacht, with a crew of six friends, also crossed the finish line in a rough weather Bermuda Race, not in first place, but not by any means the last of the 117 ships to finish. Stan further comments, "This sounds pretty self-centered, but it is the many friends I do it all with that really make it count."

As one would expect, the number of avocational interests pursued by these grown-up SRV boys far outstrips even the list of their multifaceted job descriptions. In so many ways alike and yet in so many ways so different in talents and skills, these creative individualists indicate that they are most likely to spend their time on sports that stress specific personal interest rather than intensive competition. In their apple orchard school days everybody played baseball and soccer enthusiastically. "Susie Smith was the best third baseman I have ever played with!" recalled one college professor. A couple of men still enjoy coaching junior soccer teams. Interest may be there among the men for the most popular of American sports (football, baseball, and basketball) but they are scarcely alluded to in their responses. On the other hand, outdoor activities loom large: scuba diving, tennis, fishing, travel, skiing, soaring and flying, bird watching, and gardening. Indoor interests include such things as collecting stamps or coins, repairing watches, clocks, and cameras, ship model building, carpentry, singing and instrumental music, dancing, painting, and sculpture, photography, squash and handball, acting, auto maintenance, household repair, small appliance repair, and generally "fixing things." This list is probably reflective of the general population of which these men are representative (see Introduction, page xxii), but such pursuits give collective as well as individual flavor to choices.

In their ranking of the most important factor in their lives, "My family!" was most frequently and enthusiastically ranked first, although there was no specific item in the questionnaire which called for such a response. It is a pervasive topic in the responses which are replete with emphatic adjectives and detail. In many families, interests and hobbies are shared in large measure by both partners with children and now grandchildren. Depending on family size and economic realities, the family can participate in different levels of backpacking, wilderness camping, and/or museum tours, whether these outings are close by or far away. Sometimes the parents enjoyed activities with the whole family while also maintaining their own specialities. For example, Ray says with pride, "Of course we each like coming home with blue ribbons from time to time, but hers are from beautiful paintings in art shows while mine are from sometimes crossing the line first in a sailing race. I feel more at home with a hammer or a wrench than with a watercolor brush. She's a real artist, and she plans to go right on teaching after I retire next December."

MAKING THINGS

It has often been said that "language is half of what makes us human and making tools to make things is the other half." In other words, "To engineer is human," and so it is not surprising that a large part of the group, regardless of their language facility, like to make things. Several men stretched this idea to include gardens. That the love of making things should properly pervade holistic education was the intent of the SRV curriculum design. Fortuitously, this curricular offering was particularly advantageous to the dyslexics in the group.

Edward Rawson provided a setting for many of these students to make things and explore the possibilities of the three-dimensional world. "Mister" introduced woodworking to SRV, having started a similar program in Brooklyn, NY, early in this century. Mister's concept was simple: teach each child what he needed to know at his point of development in order to build what that youngster wanted. Several of the study's members, particularly Ralph and Mark, made fully operational objects which are still in use today. Simon, the economist, has executed beautiful cabinetwork and furniture, which is still in use in his parents' living room. As late as the 1989 survey, he still mentions it as a favorite avocation.

WORKING WITH NUMBERS

Skills are taught, formulations are thought, and each helps the other. The responses to "Do you enjoy working with figures?" were apt to be clear-cut whenever likes and dislikes were expressed. A taste for mathematics undoubtedly influenced the answer as to whether one actually liked working with figures or not. Of course, it is not only talents for reading and math that differ but several other fundamental parts of intelligence. Mathematics is a language of quantity and relationships in the real and hypothetical worlds. In calculation and memory for symbols our subjects' competence closely parallels the verbal skills of reading and writing. Mathematical reasoning was seldom a problem even when the respondents were uncomfortable with calculation. Figures were often involved in such central purposes as business information, financial affairs, and scientific research. Some people, like eulexic Douglas, reported really enjoying both mathematical thinking and arithmetic practice and had fun exercising them just as he found pleasure in reading and writing. Others, like Chester, as often happens with dyslexics, suffered through calculations (with unhappy memories of multiplication tables) for the sake of pursuing their respective practical purposes. They are the ones who now thank electronic calculators for relieving anxiety and tedium.

SPEAKING AND WRITING

We explored both speaking and writing as expressive forms of verbal language. Some people like to speak in public while others do not, and some people are more or less loquacious in conversation while others tend toward silence. Sometimes fluency depends on temperament, and sometimes it may be the ability to call up and correctly pronounce words to express a specific idea or thought. Writing (penmanship or composition) is often another high hurdle between thought and expression. When asked to take a leadership role, Ray, a very dyslexic extrovert, says he would rather be president of a community organization, make speeches, and run meetings than be the secretary who must record minutes and read them aloud. In contrast, Dan's easy handwriting allows him to pay attention to what is going on and take minutes at the same time. Many penmanship problems persist and prove an additional impediment to clear and easy expression of thoughts. In one rather terse but well-expressed response, the dyslexic Frank, a competent executive, said, "I could tell you a lot more if you were right here, but writing it all out is just too hard!" In office dictation he fluently bypasses both handwriting and spelling. Sid said, "I have never learned script. I still use the manuscript lettering taught at SRV, and I actually write as little as possible and do it badly, but it's mostly legible." In another case our educational administrator, Eric, explained, "The printing above is for clarity since I normally use script!" All of the dyslexics have learned to read with understanding, and write at least passably. Each, however, complained with varying degrees of emphasis, regret, or resignation about his poor spelling, or at least expressed insecurity about its dependability. While reading may come first to mind, many aspects of the language function can tax the equanimity of even the most capable dyslexic.

The balance of freedom and discipline of the entire SRV learning experience helped to make later fulfillment possible. Half a century later, these matured skills and motivations are brought to mind by Sherman, the dyslexic medical school professor, in his brief yet modestly self-assured questionnaire answer. He said of reading, writing, and speaking in public, "I enjoy reading and regularly do so for pleasure. Speaking and writing are, of course, part of my work. I don't particularly enjoy either, but I do take a lot of satisfaction in both when I feel I've done them well." He also expressed appreciation for the tutoring which enabled him to do all of this with relative ease.

ENJOYMENT OF READING

The enjoyment of reading, instilled by the SRV experience, in these men's lives has special significance in the outcome of this study. The school's small library had specialized in interesting and challenging books of historical and scientific fiction which could often enliven, and sometimes substitute for, the more didactic textbook and encyclopedic resources in curricular studies. Such books as the *Winged Girl of Knossos, Two Children of Tyre, Little Magic Painter* (remembered by Justin) and even many of the folk and nursery tales enlarged horizons and became launching pads for lifelong interest. The men's constant exposure in childhood to good literature stimulated and encouraged their enthusiasm for reading as a form of enjoyment. Young Ralph, who came as a nonreader in third grade, had read everything there was to read about the sea by sixth grade. He became the school's authority on naval history, and built his own sextant in the school's shop. At 60, he says he sometimes still uses it when sailing.

Justin [I] was another example of SRV's holistic educational approach. He was the quiet, sensitive boy who was much more aware of the things that were important in making his school life happy than we realized. He nostalgically recalled "no teasing or bullying," but just the right mixture of aggressive play. In 1990, he recounted in detail: bird walks, campfire breakfast, and his happy participation in all that went on. Clearly eulexic he remembers many of the books of his childhood by name, and in detail, even those read aloud during rest periods after lunch so many years ago. Of course not everyone became the bookseller's ideal bibliophile like Justin, who revels in his personal library of over 4,500 volumes. When he isn't working in his wood shop, building a house, fighting developers' excesses, or backpacking, Justin has no trouble finding a good book with which to entertain his mind and spirit.

The Ph.D. sociologist, Lee [I], moderately dyslexic, after a long period of tutoring, says, "I fell in love with books and learning and have not gotten over it to this day." That all these men, even the most dyslexic of them, learned to read is a matter of record. What use do they make of this accomplishment? Success in school and in their work gives a utilitarian answer. Although the dyslexic men almost universally regretted that they could not read as fast as they would find useful, or pleasurable in some cases, in the questionnaires of 1986 and 1990 all the responses indicated that their reading skills were adequate for both comprehension and enjoyment, with interest rather than levels of difficulty determining their choices. Among the responses from the study's 44 men, only two (one eulexic and one dyslexic) said they did not really enjoy reading. Some, being slow readers, regretfully found little time to indulge in nonprofessional reading. "Everyone has the right not to read," we were once told. The answer is, "True, but one can exercise that right as an option only if he is able to read." All of these men, even the most dyslexic, have been free to choose.

Our subjects usually left their student days at SRV as competent, very often avid, readers, but this was not universally the case even with the multisensory, multimodal, and specialized tutoring provided to each student wherever needed and possible. Sometimes it was only after we had waited a long time that we saw a result that surely had our mark on its beginnings, as it was with Frank and Adam. Years ago we heard the wise SRV principal say to a parent, who was frantic about a different kind of crisis, "Of course, you don't want to just sweep this under the rug, but you can afford to be a little more tranquil about it. You know, life will teach your youngster a lot of things; you don't have to do it all, and not necessarily right now."

When our recent questionnaire asked, "do you enjoy reading?" Frank's answer was an emphatic "Yes, now!" Here is the history behind the exclamation point. In the current narrative we have been meeting Frank as the successful banker and financier who finds his most significant satisfaction in his family life and his five "great" children. When we go back to his childhood, we remember that he had reluctantly entered SRV in fifth grade, propelled by his parents' anxiety about his severe scholastic failure. In his SRV record folder we found this note from an early tutoring session: "Today Frank said, pleasantly enough, 'Why do I have to come to you for reading? My reading satisfies me.'" Still, he kept coming because it was part of his required program. Frank graduated from preparatory school and a liberal arts college, and remembers his language reeducation with appreciation. However, he says, "Except for business necessity I never opened a book after I left college until one summer when my wife and I were running a book sale for some good cause or another and something suddenly clicked—a novel caught my eye. Since then I've been reading all sorts of things just for pleasure." When the desire came, the option was open, for he knew how to read.

Adam's late-blooming, or delayed achievement of linguistic facility, is quite a different story (see page 56). He had attended SRV since nursery school, had been a rather quiet, sweet child, well-liked by his schoolmates and appropriately obliging with adults. He was shy at school, though normally active and participative at home. Adam was late in reaching developmental milestones in ways that even then seemed to this author to be perhaps neurologically significant. She was his tutor, and both had worked diligently during their many sessions together, but with discouragingly meager results in linguistic achievement by the time Adam went to another school after fourth grade. During the transition period Dr. Samuel Orton saw the boy as a patient. The author, in profound discouragement, also consulted Dr. Orton, feeling that with Adam she had failed significantly. Dr. Orton reassured her as to the boy's essential emotional intactness and made a prediction that was later benignly fulfilled. Dr. Orton pointed out that the school as a whole, as well as the tutoring, had allowed Adam to be unharmed by adverse responses to his immature behavior patterns, such as he might have suffered elsewhere. Dr. Orton felt that at some future time an appropriately knowledgeable teacher might be able to reactivate the results of his training. Adam had actually learned more than he was then able to use. Dr. Orton was certain that someday, when his development permitted, Adam could make the necessary connections to conscious awareness. Those who supervised Adam's education attempted, in various ways, to give him what he needed. Adam went through a good many years of frustration until his junior year in prep school when his mentors found a tutor whom Anna Gillingham said was one of her best graduates. With this tutor's skillful help, Adam received his diploma and went on to an excellent university where he majored in his preferred subject, American literature. Since the receipt of his B.A. degree he has had a satisfying career as a teacher of English. Dr. Orton would have been more delighted than surprised by this result.

Perhaps the experiences of Frank and Adam exemplify what Dr. Orton meant by the phrase he used several times in his speaking and writing, "the physiological habit of use." Their training had been the infrastructure, neurologically ingrained, that stood both Frank and Adam in good stead when the right time came for each one of them.

Persistent determination can sustain a dyslexic student through a long period of slow growth, as evidenced by one of the Stanford Achievement Test records (standard administration) from the SRV files. There was very slow but consistently steady improvement in year-end scores. Barely up to grade level by age twelve but conscious of his own needs, Dan was reported in high school to be a cheerful hard worker "and a popular student leader, too." Dan told the author that whenever he could manage it, he elected the English courses with the "hardest" teachers because they seemed to have the most to teach him about what he knew he needed to learn. In law school he declined being editor-in-chief of his year's Law Review because he was more interested in the writing practice he would gain as case editor of that publication. Such determined planning has surely played a part in Dan's slow but steadily accelerating climb up the ladder of success recounted in Chapter 7. In his 1990 questionnaire he says generously to his appreciative tutor, "Thank you for all you have done for me. Without your initial help and encouragement I couldn't, and wouldn't, have achieved to the extent I have." His tutor, however, recognizes that a major factor in the successful outcome is Dan's consistent steadfastness in holding himself to his own values and purposes.

PERSISTENCE OF PERSONALITY PATTERNS

The high self-consistency among our dyslexic and nondyslexic subjects shows in their growth from early childhood to late maturity. Dan's steady, thoughtful, persistent, rational, innovative determination was observed in preschool years. If we next review his whole school and personality history, we should not be surprised that the result is a competent lawyer, who became a manufacturer, a businessman, an investment counselor, and a community leader, whose judgment everyone has continuously trusted and whose company all still enjoy.

Patrick, who chuckles over the memory of his ingenious youth when he found ways to plunge the school into temporary darkness, helped turn his electronics interest into a career. His sense of mischievous humor has helped him maintain a good rapport with the troubled youths with whom he now works and counsels in electronics clubs. He spends much of his time and effort organizing constructive outlets for the technological ingenuity and interests of these boys so they need not become social misfits and can enjoy life in the late twentieth century.

Overcoming difficulties is something people such as these men learn to do at an early age. Pursuing various hobbies and accomplishing solid professional work can be equally satisfying. And so the hyperactivity, which is hard for adults to cope with in children, can produce an effective and interesting adult when it is appropriately controlled.

People manifest such a variety of interweaving and overlapping traits that it is difficult to categorize individuals into subtypes however convincingly one can arrange their characteristics into categories or items in a logical outline. Seen in this light the persistence of influences and adaptational talents related to dyslexia are more readily understandable and acceptable as part of the way things are in life, not something strange with a kind of pathological etiology.

ON BEING DYSLEXIC

It was commonly recognized among the boys during school years that some people needed a lot of help in intensive tutoring, some a little, and some none at all, and that one progressed and, after while, usually "graduated from tutoring." It was one of the things you might have to do, but in today's idiom, it was "no big deal." Tutoring was talked about, but not pejoratively. The boys and their families were ahead of the public opinion of that time, and were still ahead of it in both knowledge and attitudes when we saw one another in 1965. With dyslexia much more in the public eye in 1990, I wondered how they felt about being classified in that way.

We know from the records and later reports that most of the boys had become competent in language skills during their elementary school years, whatever their innate endowments. The few who had not yet "made the grade" in the pertinent skills or beyond levels that would satisfy their ultimate purposes continued to progress until they did so, like Frank. By 1990 the dyslexics among them had settled, albeit somewhat regretfully, for reading speeds slower than they desired. Some had discovered degrees of ineptitude in such areas as foreign language learning, higher mathematical notation, and organization of verbal thinking and abstraction. Of the remaining insufficiencies, as in spelling and sometimes in handwriting, they seemed to have accepted dyslexia as a probable reason but by no means an excuse for inadequate performance in some areas. In their responses to the demands of language they seemed, often quite consciously, to be "in charge and glad of it," capable of enjoying "the examined life" when they chose to be reflective.

In reports, interviews, or informal conversations (as at the anniversary celebration at SRV in 1989), the subject of dyslexia and the men's involvement in it was open to a sort of interested, free, and easy discussion that seemed rather casual. This attitude is in stark contrast to the tension that commonly accompanies references in the wider culture, either in a discussion of the problem as a whole or in the acceptance by those who have succeeded the hard way against severe odds. The common motto, *per aspera ad astra* (through difficulties to the stars), may be their route, but the SRV men have demonstrated that achievement need not be accompanied by psychological scar tissue. In fact, the quality of their lives has actually been enhanced not only by their acceptance of themselves but also by the whole idea of dyslexia and its occurrence among their friends, relatives, and offspring. This has led to a more comfortable feeling of competence in meeting the needs of those for whom they are responsible, as with Frank and his son or eulexic Everett and his adopted dyslexic son.

As we follow the men, they continue to report slow reading, poor spelling, and sometimes other difficulties, as did Roger recently adding, "but people like us have to recognize our limitations and figure out how to do what we want to do in spite of them." To be sure, this could be said of any of us, but there are some deficiencies of talent that can be disregarded with relative impunity. In a literate, technological culture like ours, however, it is the very limitations of which Roger is speaking whose pivotal importance demand adaptation. It has been heartening to see the many ways in which this generally high-functioning group of men have met their challenges, managing not to sacrifice much but often to enrich the quality of their lives.

Chapter IX

THIS STUDY AND THE FIELD OF DYSLEXIA

THE FIELD OF DYSLEXIA

In this chapter some questions previously acknowledged but not re-
solved can now be addressed with more confidence because of further
experience, new knowledge, and much research over the past half-century. Of particular relevance have been studies in neurobiology and evolution, genetics and linguistics, and clinical psychology and evaluation.
Considering our previously insufficiently addressed questions in light of
the newer insights should make the facts and events shown in our composite case histories more germane and may further illuminate the connection of our study with broader generalizations in the whole field. This
new knowledge has given us welcome assurance of the reasonableness of
our educational treatment, while at the same time raising more questions
about the underlying systems at work in each individual.

DEFINITION

The question of a definition for the term of "dyslexia" must be addressed. There are some concepts, like language itself, of which it can be
said that everybody knows what it is, but no one has been able to present
a wholly satisfactory definition of it. Experience has convinced me that
dyslexia is such a concept. The best that one can do in such a case is to
name what one is talking about and then describe it with an appropriate
explanatory purpose or viewpoint. One such view might be the center of
interest of the describer, while another could be an attempt to cast the

description into the verbal language comfortable to one's respondent, whether colleague or audience.

Specific definitions of dyslexia have been offered, and some have even gained widespread approval. Let us look at three such formulations which are pertinent here. Each one at its time and in its way arose from somewhere close to the center of the field of dyslexia.

As it happened, at exactly the time of publication of The School in Rose Valley study in 1968, Macdonald Critchley, M.D., president of the World Federation of Neurology, called together the Federation's ad hoc Committee on Dyslexia. This committee consisted of leaders of several disciplines of the neurosciences and came from many countries around the world. After some days of deliberation its members agreed upon the following definition, which has since been widely used:

> Developmental Dyslexia: A disorder manifested by difficulty in learning to read despite conventional instruction, adequate intelligence, and socio-cultural opportunity. It is dependent upon fundamental cognitive disabilities which are frequently of constitutional origin.

Of this definition Dr. Critchley himself said, "Although not perfect, it is a good working definition. . . . 'Developmental dyslexia' subsumes more than a mere problem with reading; it constitutes a veritable syndrome of language-impairments." This explication of the word "reading" makes the World Federation of Neurology's point of view and the experiences represented by The School in Rose Valley study coincide.

In 1994 the Research Committee of the Orton Dyslexia Society felt the need for a newer working definition of dyslexia in scientific terms as precisely focused as was possible on current research needs. It proposed, and the Board of Directors of the Society accepted, the following as a position statement, subject to review and whatever modifications or clarifications are necessary. The explication of the exact use of each term is beyond the scope of this chapter but helps to clarify to nonscientists such usages as "single word decoding." Again, as in the World Federation of Neurology's definition, this formulation is suitable for its purposes. It more clearly focuses on fundamental work and is still commensurate with the findings of The School in Rose Valley study and conclusions from related fields of practice. The Orton Dyslexia Society Research Committee's definition of 1994 is:

> Dyslexia is one of several distinct learning disabilities. It is a specific language-based disorder of constitutional origin characterized by difficulties

in single word decoding, usually reflecting insufficient phonological processing abilities. These difficulties in single word decoding are often unexpected in relation to age and other cognitive and academic abilities; they are not the result of generalized developmental disability or sensory impairment. Dyslexia is manifested by variable difficulty with different forms of language, often including, in addition to problems with reading, a conspicuous problem with acquiring proficiency in writing and spelling.

This sharply targeted attempt to isolate unique identifying characteristics of the named syndrome is important in light of its research purposes and adds measurably to our understanding of much that we have observed in our study. However, by its nature, it necessarily gives short shrift to certain skills, attributes, and traits that may be integral or peripheral but are frequently encountered parts of the pattern we call dyslexia.

In response to requests from its membership, the president of the International Orton Dyslexia Society appointed a special society-wide committee to craft a more general definition. The committee's mandate was to obtain the views which represented the Society's entire constituency as widely as possible. This included all levels of interest, background, and modalities of approach from the leaders and advisors of long standing and high expertise to those of the youngest, newest, and least sophisticated members involved in the problems associated with dyslexia. This definition is more inclusive or global in nature, and is designed to answer the question, "What is the dyslexia we are talking about?" Ideally, it should be offered by a spokesperson who is familiar with the concept's central pattern and its many possible ramifications as experienced by the questioner and rephrased or interpreted in language comfortably familiar to that questioner. The resulting general purpose definition, adopted at the Society's annual meeting in November, 1994, reads as follows:

Dyslexia is a neurologically-based, often familial, disorder which interferes with the acquisition and processing of language. Varying in degrees of severity, it is manifested by difficulties in receptive and expressive language, including phonological processing, in reading, writing, spelling, handwriting, and sometimes in arithmetic. Dyslexia is not a result of lack of motivation, sensory impairment, inadequate instructional or environmental opportunities, or other limiting conditions, but may occur together with these conditions. Although dyslexia is lifelong, individuals with dyslexia frequently respond successfully to timely and appropriate intervention.

Obviously, 26 years have not put full agreement into words, but equally obvious is the scientific temper reflected in the willingness to use carefully considered statements so that collaboration may go on until still better attempts can be forged.

Socrates, 2400 years ago, noted that any reputed expert, pushed into a corner for an exact definition in his home territory, had finally to extricate himself by giving a case instance, analogue, or metaphor. I believe the philosopher would be subject to that same experience were he to foregather with a body of present-day "experts" in the field of dyslexia. Linguists call such terms radial concepts, concepts which go out from their centers in all directions. Our present situation, I think, gives evidence of life and growth, however aggravating it may be to some seekers of exactitude.

Socrates might now find the most succinct expression of the term dyslexia to be that of Alfred, a real boy whom I have quoted many times, since 1965 (compare with the footnote on page 3). Al, the person most involved at the true center of the dyslexia domain, said, "I can think OK. What's wrong is just my words. I forget them, and I can't manage them." The further realities described in The School in Rose Valley inquiry should speak to the mind of today's most insistent Socratic questioner.

The concept of the field of dyslexia as an entity has a rich foundation in its history and precursors in neurobiological science which can be seen clearly in the work of the field's first major 20th century synthesizer, Samuel T. Orton. Following the lead of Hinshelwood in 1896 and his 1917 text, Orton's global outline of the scope and logic of dyslexia were brought together in 1925, and developed by him and his associates in the next two decades. The essential outline of the viewpoint was described in the early chapters of Part I of this volume and provides the theoretical and empirical background of the study here concluded. Being aware of the many roads that it might have been possible to take, I had surveyed, and in many cases, explored and drawn material from other avenues of approach to language problems by 1965–68, but had found the Orton approach to be for me a rational and effective core. Over the ensuing years I have continued to investigate other avenues and wherever they looked promising, I tried them, incorporating from them what seemed useful. As this study draws to a close, I am satisfied and feel that experience has validated such a course.

Dr. Orton considered "specific language disability," now called dyslexia, not to be a categorically definable disease, like measles or malaria, or an organic deficit, such as a missing limb or organ. He viewed it, from the long evolutionary perspective, as related to the latest and, hence, the least finished faculty in the development of the human species and in each of its members. The coexisting difficulties and advantages of such a stage of development are the components of adaptation, growth, and selectively reinforced change which is the core of Darwinian evolution and also of the life sequence development of each individual.

Roger Saunders (psychologist and nationally known leader in the diagnosis and treatment of dyslexia) and I have previously written that in the field of dyslexia "the differences are personal; the diagnosis, clinical; the treatment, educational; and the understanding, scientific and empathetic." So far in this study we have considered chiefly the diagnostic and educational aspects and have seen the personal differences among the men. We next turn to what we know about language and language functioning; how the new findings in scientific knowledge enlighten this study; and, how this study may contribute to the development of scientific knowledge.

In our society, severe reading disability has generally been, and still usually is, the starting point of acute interest in the field of dyslexia. It is as the circle of involvement widens that the whole of language learning becomes focal and its many manifestations show their connections with the interfacing disciplines which inform the field. The "dyslexia generalist," as I have come to describe myself, needs to explore as many areas of this domain as possible, while recognizing the nature and value of the special interests and contributions of those with different centers.

The severely dyslexic person may be seen at first glance as an anomaly when it comes to language functioning. However, my work and that of others in the field has led me to see that person—as Orton did—near the extreme end of a language acquisition dimension with the eulexic at the other end. Between the two poles are many people who may experience either little or no problem with language, while others exhibit some, most, or all of the constellation of traits we have associated with the syndrome of dyslexia.

SCIENCE AND THE FIELD OF DYSLEXIA

Among the scientists to whom I feel most indebted are previously mentioned neurologists such as Richard L. Masland for his wisdom and vision in the field of dyslexia, Macdonald Critchley for his unflinching commitment to the exploration of the nature of the language function, and Norman Geschwind for his versatile and creative explanation of neuronal processing and functioning. My understanding has also been increased by Albert Galaburda's description of the neuroanatomical structure of the brain from many angles, especially in dyslexic individuals, and Martha Denckla's recognition of people's versatility of talents as well as an understanding of the highest levels of language organizational skill requiring pragmatic judgment and controlled flexibility which she calls the "executive function." Paula Tallal's blended theoretical and humane interest in the very young child, Margaret Livingstone's study of neurocellular processing rates, and Christiana Leonard's exploration of noninvasive imaging of the cortical structure of the brains of dyslexic and nondyslexic individuals have all added to my insights as has Thomas G. West's consideration of visual processing in the light of modern technology. In addition, Gerald Edelman, immunologist and neuroscientist, has given me a conceptual framework in which to analyze information I had previously understood in a more limited context.

Deepened insights into genetics and its connection with evolution and the present questions of familial inheritance have reached me particularly through the work of Hallgren, Sladen, Vandenberg, De Fries, and Pennington. Shankweiler and the Libermans have been among my most directly personal connections with psycholinguistics. Other people and their work have been most helpful, the list and the literature of which I can only allude to. What is important here is the light they have shed on what came to me out of the SRV experience, my private practice, and other professional pursuits.

These scientists' conclusions also seem to underscore the rationale and practice of the Orton-Gillingham approach to the teaching of language to all learners, but especially to those who are constitutionally or factually dyslexic. Bias admitted, this explanation for the success of this methodology with a long and intensively studied sample, is deeply satisfying.

PATTERNS OF INHERITANCE

The genetic process we are talking about is, of course, the old story of heredity retold in the light of new understanding. The more we learn about the nature of our genes and their diversity, the more we must realize what neophytes we are. We are dazzled by the complexity of the long development of animal life, including our own, and the antiquity and underlying structure of any language we learn. Inheritance has made itself felt in our SRV men among whose families there have appeared many of the diverse patterns of talents and difficulties that my practice and the experience of colleagues the world-over know as dyslexia.

GENETICS AND FAMILIAL HERITABILITY

Observers have long recognized the importance of the familial component in differences in language-learning facility, and I raised this question in several places in Part I, but much of its scientific significance was still unproven in 1968. Now we have much more information which we can apply to our study.

Previously, we had seen familial patterns of dyslexia between generations, but the various studies of twins—from Hallgren (1950) to Pennington (lecture, 1994)—show that the fundamental etiology of dyslexia is significantly genetic. These studies of identical and fraternal twins compared to nontwin siblings and nonrelated persons show how strong the genetic link is to the presence of dyslexia. Environment obviously plays a part in the manifestations and such interaction of inheritance and environment is an example of the interplay of nature and nurture.

Do the questions of heritability and the SRV longitudinal study throw any light on each other? We have looked at the original subjects in Part I as well as in Chapters 7 and 8, and often reflect upon their parents as well. However, we are often asked about their children. In the latter case, for instance in the lowest of the original three language groups (LLF III), four examples of obvious likeness occur in father and child pairs. In the case of these pairs, recent tests by competent examiners have brought forth reports which almost sound as if they might have been written years ago about the children's father, as we will see in some examples below.

Not all dyslexics have dyslexic children, and not all other children in the families of the above pairs are rated dyslexic. It is often this way in connection with a condition made up of many components. Case material taken from inheritance patterns in this group give real life examples of such interconnections; now in diagnosis we can use this material with much less hesitancy than was expressed in our 1968 analysis.

Sometimes when we look afresh at our subjects' parents' generation, a single factor stands out. For example, when Dan was about ten and his brother, Eric, was eight, back in the 1940's, their charming, intelligent mother, Carla, was at work on a post-master's course in reading in order to understand better the work her sons were doing in multisensory language instruction. One insight she had gained was shown when she told the boys' tutor (this author), "You know, I believe these boys are just like their mother!" The speaking and listening experiences she related validated her judgment. So seldom do we have a sharply focused self-analytical account of a single sensory phenomenon that her story is worth recounting in detail. She said, "When I hear someone speak, it takes me much longer to get the idea from here (pointing to her ear) to here (pointing to the top of her head) than it does other people. I have to sit in the front row in class and watch the professor every moment or I lose track of his words, miss the connection and get all mixed up . . . When we have guests and someone tells a hilarious joke, the conversation goes on and my belated laughter makes everyone stare at me, and I feel so foolish!" I brought her problem to the attention of Dr. Ralph Preston, my colleague (see page v), who was her professor. Dr. Preston told me that her intensity of attention was disconcerting, but it relieved him to understand its cause. Although the details differed between mother and sons, all experienced a similar language problem to a greater or lesser degree.

Carla's sons, both in our LLF Group III, reported several decades later that things were linguistically well with their own now grown-up children, "except for one modest speech defect"—the kind of thing that seems to run in the mother's family. Of course, family members' language traits are never "just alike," however recognizably similar they maybe. The British neurologist Macdonald Critchley (Critchley and Critchley, 1978) said "the syndrome of developmental dyslexia contains enough minor variations to make nearly every case a clinical collector's item." If we knew a wider circle of Dan's and Eric's relatives, we might find that the whole family had a more diversified pattern, but in the representatives of the three generations we do know, it has been problems with the spoken language that have made trouble for them. Inadequacies in listening and speaking, despite normal hearing and high intelligence, are commonly recognized as precursors to reading and spelling problems as they were with Dan and Eric.

Every person and family included in this study is in some measure a part of its totality, but the "second family" briefly described in Chapter 4 (see pages 100–101) seems quintessentially typical of the study's population. Facts drawn from the life histories of its boys, here known as Jerry, Harvey, and Jasper, illustrate in one family some aspects of the complex diversity of heritability in the field of dyslexia as I have observed it.

Jerry, severely dyslexic himself, reports that all three of his children are "dyslexic to some degree." Both daughters responded well to childhood tutoring; both have earned master's degrees and are special-needs teachers, as was Jerry at their age. Jerry's son, "not a student" but apparently possessing visual talent, is an artist, and attended art school for two years. Jerry, in his SRV school days, is remembered as a witty, clever and facile cartoonist.

In the mid-60's Harvey's fifth grade son gave the author, on a brief SRV visit, a startling illusion of time-travel. There, but for a generation's passage, was Jerry—his uncle—a twin in appearance, movement, and scholastics. In the 1990 study Harvey wrote that this son had had "some reading problems, but no diagnosis" and was owner and manager of a retail business at 35 with a B.A. degree. No language difficulties are mentioned among his other children. Harvey is a medical scientist and university administrator to whom all things academic have always been extremely easy. He says of his brothers, "Yes I can do those [scholastic] things, but it is Jerry and Jasper who sparkle." I have always thought that Harvey, too, has plenty of "sparkle." We notice, however, Harvey's strong left laterality, an orientation often found in families with a dyslexic predisposition. The correlation between dyslexia and laterality is in dispute, but my experience has indicated a connection between the two.

Jerry and Harvey still live near The School in Rose Valley and are very much a part of its community. Their younger brother Jasper, who lives in New York State, draws from the same gene pool. Jasper says, "of course I'm dyslexic even though you don't say so in the book and so are both the kids; one an auditory type and the other a visual type. You even have the psychologist's report to prove it with Drew." Drew's grandmother (Jasper's mother) had told me years earlier, "This child is not flourishing and we wonder why?" Jasper and his wife were referred to a New York psychologist who made Drew's diagnosis. The three mens' father, their paternal uncle, and some relatives of the next degree in both parents' families had had significant reading difficulties.

Paralleling Jasper's case there are several instances of parent-child similarities which suggest inheritance of dyslexic characteristics. For example, there was Ralph, who brought his nine-year-old son Warren, to me for testing, saying, "He seems so much like me at the same age." Test results supported the father's observations, both then and later, as Warren went on through school to a university degree and a job in business. Meanwhile, Warren's younger brother and sister have chosen two quite different career paths and have no apparent dyslexia problems. The sister has received a master's degree in English, and the brother has pursued a career in business. Meanwhile, their mother has become a highly trained tutor of dyslexic children. This one family shows several of the patterns of inheritance observed among others in the SRV series. Those who like to follow case history trails may want to go back to Ralph's childhood as the boy of the "third family" described in Chapter 4, pages 101–102.

Another of the men, Angus, also asked me to test his elder daughter, Andrea, then in third grade. During the evaluation she misspelled her own name in two different ways and made other errors which substantiated Angus' suspicion that she had some problems. On his later questionnaire Angus volunteered that all three of his children are "dyslexic . . . just like me."

Frank, the banker, now a financial advisor, has three college-graduate daughters. His older son, Gregory, under parental pressure, finished high school but never liked school. Frank reports that "there was no identified LD (learning disability), but now I wonder!" (See Chapter 8.) Frank's younger son, Milton, five years Greg's junior, received help at a school for children with learning disabilities where Frank then became an active, well-informed parent. At the time of the 1990 study, Milton was attending a college designed for dyslexics, still finding it difficult to get his ideas into written form although the college reported him to be a very hard working student. A psychologist's recent report assessing his good intelligence and other characteristics could almost describe the Frank remembered from The School in Rose Valley. Along with the report was a recent writing sample quite indicative of a severely dyslexic person.

Frank's ". . . but now I wonder!" comment is an item of hindsight which calls to mind a component of the SRV culture. We have noticed instances elsewhere in the histories of Jasper, Ray, Ralph, Angus, Dan and Eric, Everett, and other parents who either "wondered," knew, or perhaps recognized the connection between some of their children's characteristics and their own childhood experiences. When our subjects were schoolboys, it was the business of the adults to be conscious of clinical diagnoses and the pedagogy of treatment. For the children it was still proper that any recognized differences should be personal. We were glad to have them think of themselves as "regular guys who were having some schoolwork problems that their elders were bothered about." Maybe (as with Frank) this assistance was a nuisance, but with others it was recognized as necessary and helpful or "no big deal." Their self esteem was minimally affected unless we were dealing with the after-effects of previous failure.

When, in turn, the boys in the original study became parents, each was likely first to interpret what he saw in his own children in the light of his own remembered childhood. Whether in clinically diagnosed cases or in anecdotally reported instances, the 1990 reports of the new generation reflect both heritable language patterns and sources of parental attitudes. For instance in Ray's family, as in Ralph's, three children have drawn from the family's collection of traits. "Ray, Jr." looks almost exactly like the boy we used to know so well in the '40's, but it is one of the two girls whose academic hardships her father described as "much like mine, but not as bad." Like her more academically inclined siblings, she has graduated from a four-year liberal arts college, and welcomes the challenges of her vigorous life as a park ranger and environmentalist who enjoys cross-country bicycling with friends.

In the case material secondary to our 1965 and 1990 reports we saw other familial likenesses. The younger brothers of Mark, Nicholas, Luke, and Roger, all known clinically to the author but not in the study, had especially severe language-learning problems. The younger brothers succeeded academically and vocationally with appropriate tutorial help, personal motivation, and special school and family support. In 1990, they were engaged as an engineer, two university professors, and a high school English teacher. This was further supportive of, and in line with, the documented cases of their older dyslexic brothers.

EVOLUTION AND HUMAN DEVELOPMENT

At any animal's conception, evolution has gone far with genes and inherited tendencies towards projecting what the individual will become in accordance with the species' "master plan." Environment has also played a part as the individual becomes a recognizable member of the species during its embryonic period. The constancy factor is set by the form and function that determine the limits within which a species is, in fact, a species. This leaves room at the growing edges for the variations which allow for the uniqueness of each individual.

Nowhere is this more amazingly shown than with respect to the emergence of language, the most recent and humanly species-specific characteristic. When the human child is born, anywhere on earth, he/she comes into life at the exquisitely right stage for language acquisition, with every organ and potential "at the ready." The infant is not yet speaking, understanding speech, or even able to make controlled, let alone meaningful, gestures. The child needs a long childhood in a surrounding culture, with its support and stimuli, in which to become a separate self. So there must be a connecting bridge which the senses will provide.

To use another metaphor: with each person, life weaves a fabric with the warp set by genetics, evolution, and heredity. The shuttle is partly loaded in the embryonic stage, added to during gestation, and comes to birth open for the next contribution of environmental yarn. Some of its thread is already there in terms of built-in developmental Jacquard-like "patterning" of age-related developments that are to come. The exact continuation will depend on circumstances and culture, the sources of almost infinite variation in the color and texture in the yarn on the shuttle. The child is just able enough and just unfinished enough to take for its own the ways and the speech patterns of the surrounding human world to which he/she is exposed. Evolution has given such a "neat" package that we can but marvel.

Redundancy in nature is necessary for the survival of species, so obvious in the millions of "unused" seeds and eggs, and gives opportunity to the variations essential for evolution to take place. It should, then, not surprise us to find redundancy in the psycho-neurological structures and processes in that most complex of nature's phenomena, the human brain.

In the connection between self and reality there is a necessary minimum of sensory bridging early in life, dramatically exemplified by the opening up of the symbolic world to deaf and blind Helen Keller. As a child working with her teacher, Ann Sullivan, Helen discovered that the matter she was touching gave a delightful sensation, and if spelled into her hand had a name. That opened a floodgate to everything else. From that point on she quickly developed a facility and mastery of language, which many people believed rested on an extraordinary sense of touch. At Miss Keller's request, Samuel T. Orton later tested her tactile ability and found it less than average. The point is well-taken: sensory bridging, no matter how shaky or how good, is a prerequisite in engaging one with the world of language. One does the best with what one has, for there is a strong drive to use one's symbolic capacity. Sharp, clear sensory function gives obvious advantage in language acquisition, but at points where one sense may be inadequate, another can often come to its support or can be taught to do so.

Although extremely variable in sensory abilities, none of our subjects was at Helen Keller's deprivation level, nor, as far as we know, at the exceptionally talented sensory level. The range of our LLF scale here, as elsewhere, seems to represent what Orton posited as the "range of normal neurophysiological variation," open to careful observation and realistic accommodation. Even Carla's extreme example of her inability to follow spoken language fits here, for in day-to-day conversations her limitation was scarcely apparent.

PSYCHOLINGUISTICS

For modern psycholinguistics to be useful in diagnosis and treatment one must relate the current achievement of a language learner's skills to those appropriate to his or her age, general development, and personal needs. In recent decades marked gains in both linguistic science and psychoeducational measurement have so increased understanding and test reliability as to improve significantly clinical judgments and teaching procedures and our faith in them. It seems, on the basis of the results, that Orton's scientific orientation and Gillingham and Stillman's careful scholarship, combined with the controlled flexibility that characterized their approach, had pointed our SRV efforts in a fruitful direction.

Chance, it is said, favors the prepared mind. That it may also serve the learning mind was, it has seemed to me, illustrated by my initiation into the field of dyslexia. In the education of teachers, I have noticed that it is often from their first practicum students that, by rigorous application of a good core methodology, beginners learn memorably significant lessons. In this respect I myself was doubly fortunate. In the first place, I had been taught language skills in childhood by methods quite compatible with those recommended by Orton and Gillingham.[1] They had not invented the teaching procedures but had synthesized them into an approach especially suitable to the needs of language impaired learners, one which I,

---

[1]By pure coincidence, it was in the same year, 1905, that Anna Gillingham had her first teaching job at West Philadelphia Friends School while I was in the first grade at the Girard Avenue Friends School in the same city. Our schools used a text, *New Education Readers: Book One* (Demarest & Van Sickle, 1900) which stressed what we now call the multisensory approach to learning phonics. Presumably, Gillingham used the same series, since both schools were in the same system. I realized this happenstance only while working on this text.

accordingly, found relatively easy to acquire and use, once I had been made aware of it.

Then, as it happened, my first student was Peter, whom I had known since age three. He had had almost "all the problems in the book" and was still struggling with several of them by sixth grade in 1935. Each component problem, by that time, was not excessively severe, except for his complete unawareness of phonetics, but in sum they were enough to constitute a "specific developmental language disability" of educationally crippling proportions. With a fresh start after Orton's diagnosis, I had to learn to cope not only with the residuals of Peter's agonizingly delayed and imperfect early speech and stuttering and their accompanying cyclonic behavior, but with the whole linguistic sequence of the multisensory, phonological needs of a boy with limited and distorting facility in auditory and visual memory. However, he was a most suitable subject for me as a newcomer to the field. It was remarkable that a basically well-schooled beginner, with an eager student and an appropriate teaching approach carefully followed, could achieve in eight school months a gain of four and one-half years tested growth in reading scores (to grade 7.5) as well as grade improvements in other subjects. It was hard to believe but became a matter of record. Except for unreliable spelling and for difficulty with cursive writing and the reading of it, Peter was ready to go into secondary school with his classmates. This was more rapid progress than the Ortons had predicted. Peter continued to take reading courses while in high school and college and enjoyed many kinds of literature.

Once again chance favored my education by providing as my next three dyslexic students Roger, Henry, and Jerry, whose diagnoses of specific linguistic inadequacies were made by Dr. Paul Dozier. These inadequacies had to do with verbal symbols of language only; Jerry (visual language symbols) had graphic talents, and Henry (word enunciation) had "perfect pitch" on the violin, while Roger's mild dyspraxia was general, specific-language inclusive. Seeming reasonable and certainly effective at that time, the steps that were followed by Peter and his successors now have further scientific validation from other sources as stages in psycholinguistic development. These stages are from birth to maturity: movement, gesture, or sign language; phonology with phonemic awareness and fluent spoken language; the addition of the alphabetic principle for visible language of reading and writing; orthography, the "right-writing" or spelling patterns of the language; morphology, the form and derivation of words related to their meaning; syntactic and grammatical structure, or the way the language goes together; organization and style, the more complex symbolic formulation and expression necessary for full literacy.

SRV students in the tutoring program, not only those in this study, went through as much of this sequence as their individual development, and their time and the teaching resources at the school permitted, with many linguistic results among those hitherto recounted. Peter and Jerry, for example, eventually completed doctoral dissertations, as could Henry and Roger if they had so chosen.

Once again, constancy and variation come into play. Spoken language, which is universal, requires post-natal triggering and interpersonal experience; written language, which is not universal and comes much later in the evolutionary scale, requires more specific teaching. In the cases of Peter and the others, this scheme proves out again and again. There is often to be a gap between the ability to speak and read, showing the differences of complexity and abstract processes of the spoken code and the written cipher. This change of modality from auditory to visual-auditory comes, as we have said, much later in the evolutionary scale of development, but represents an almost universal potential. Practically every child, I believe, can learn to read and write with the requisite teaching.

THE SRV LANGUAGE LEARNING FACILITY
GROUPS REVISED

Review of the Language Learning Facility Scale which was devised for our 1965 study naturally suggests some changes in classification and grouping in light of present knowledge and thought. As before, I feel most secure about the placement of individuals at the upper and lower ends of the scale. After a study of new findings in the field, including consideration of detailed reexamination of old as well as new individual records and consultation about them with several colleagues and peers, I am ready to reappraise the positions of some subjects. With continued use of the Language Learning Facility Scale as a baseline, no changes seem needed at the extremes, but the whole group can now be divided into two, rather than three, parts with 22 of the 44 men still active in the study in each classification. The rearrangements leave seventeen (all of the survivors) of the original Language Learning Facility Group III in their position as dyslexics, although their exact rank order has become less relevant. I am ready to add to their company Nicholas, Jasper, and Sid, originally rank-ordered just above the dyslexics and counted as "mildly dyslexic" but placed in a nondyslexic category (LLF II). Jasper and Sid have recently expressed that they have often felt encumbered in just such ways as have been reported by the others of the dyslexic group. Mark's move into the dyslexic category has already been discussed in Chapter 7. Dirk was identified as dyslexic in secondary school where the dyslexia was seen to have at least as much effect on his adjustment to academic demands as did his partial deafness. His placement is marginal.

In Nicholas' case, a questionable diagnosis made by an ill-informed clinical consultant demonstrates how important it is to a diagnostician to have detailed knowledge both of an individual's background and of the fundamental nature of dyslexia. In retrospect, I remember trying to stay awake after lunch while listening to Nicholas, age nine, as he painfully slowly decoded a line of very simple text for which his phonological skills were adequate but not yet at a fluency level. Nicholas had always been a frail child, and even in the fourth grade he was absent for a quarter of the school days due to minor illnesses. Nevertheless, references to Nick's contemporary records showed this to be his "wake-up year," when he was belatedly outgrowing overdependence on adult help. His language learning was far from facile, but he was now earnestly working at it because he, himself, had found a way in which he really could learn to read. None of this was known nor asked about by the clinician, who had seen the boy without consultation with the author or the school. He rated Nicholas as very intelligent, somewhat immature, not dyslexic but, he said critically, very slow at reading by reason of his dependence on phonics. Of course, we would have told him, better slow reading than no reading, for this was the way Nick was having to learn, "as fast as possible but as slowly as necessary for eventual and lasting success." Our 1965 classification of "late blooming" was made, however reluctantly, in deference to the clinical opinion. As usual, we offered transitional assistance when any student was enrolled in another school, and the principal of Nick's next school did consult with us. Fortunately, his new school was already using a classroom adaptation of our SRV phonological program and thus was able to continue approximately what we had been doing with him, though less intensively.

Nick's scholastic success was later attested to by his B.A. and M.S. degrees and his careers—first in scientific research, then shifting to computer service management and consultancy. In 1990 he reported that he very much enjoys reading but still reads "much too slowly." He still prefers a quiet environment without the confusion which often besets him in a crowded workplace or social situation, though he is at ease with individuals. Nick considers himself "mildly dyslexic," just where I had placed him on the Language Learning Facility Scale in 1965, although when I knew him as a child, I should have been more comfortable considering him as "moderately affected but with a good prognosis." Whatever the degree, Nick was, the clinician's diagnosis notwithstanding, and still is a proper member of the lower language group.

The new 1990 division puts 22 of the 44 active participants in the constitutionally dyslexic group. This is almost a watershed, but not quite clearly so. Perhaps some of these low-language talent men might have learned to read "somehow," with or without enthusiasm. It had not been our policy to delay diagnosis until failure as was common practice; we had tried to take preventative action if we saw roadblocks ahead preferring to err on the precautionary side. Also, to qualify the aspects of linguistic excellence within the nondyslexic group, there are those among the other 22 who have symptoms of language difficulty. Duncan, for example, came to the school because of his parents' concern about language and math difficulties. These were rather quickly overcome, but he is still conscious of his past and has recently discussed his possible dyslexia with me. I know of nondisabling wisps of a language problem, as in his case, in almost all the other men in the middle of the original distribution, "nondyslexic." Six of them have brothers and one a first cousin among the lower-language 22.

In the parallel consideration of the neurological and behavioral aspects of dyslexia we come back once again to the varied manifestation within the language continuum. Orton, for example, gave reasons for considering stuttering and speech dysfluencies to be neurologically connected with the other language disability symptoms. Among our subjects we were several times aware of stuttering but had found it to be generally overcome without intervention by middle childhood. However, one particularly interesting instance of speech dysfluency was that of Walt (see Part I, page 49). From very early childhood Walt was in every other way an excellent user of language. His persistent stuttering was wisely handled by his parents. During a 1964 conversation with his parents in the East while Walt was living in the Northwest, we were reminded by them of the mother's other relatives who had had severe reading problems. Nevertheless, the three of us had concluded that Walt was not dyslexic, that his stuttering came from some other undetermined source. In 1990 Walt seldom hesitated noticeably in speech, but claimed to have a dyslexic son, so perhaps we were too much influenced by his eulexic talents and should now give more weight to the heritability factor and the stuttering as indicators of dyslexia. In Walt's case his inheritance also contributes to our reappraisal, but he has been left, marginally, in the nondyslexic group.

We now have our groups rearranged in accordance with such logic and understanding as we have gained in both general and particular terms by the 1990's. Social validation (case consultations with current professional peers) has also been a valuable check, promoting objectivity in reexamining original judgments.

INCIDENCE

Ever since the days of the 1965 study I have been plagued by the question of the high incidence of dyslexia in the SRV population. I had an awareness of the very real dangers of investigator-bias, particularly in this unique situation, and addressed both that question and the incidence problem in several places in Part I (see Chapters 2 and 3, pages 7–12, and especially page 18; also pages 29–30 and 43). I think I have now found something I missed in my precautions: the self-selection factor inherent in the population matrix from which our SRV subjects were drawn.

In the first place it was, as we recognized, a private school population. The private schools in our area were not generally oriented toward specific language learning disability, but, as is usually the case, there was a higher percentage of such students than the schools recognized. Parents want help for special needs and often put this high in their family budget priorities. Secondly, and even more importantly, we acknowledged the nature of The School in Rose Valley parent group itself. These were independent thinkers, not only with a high tolerance for diversity but with a strong value orientation toward such individual differences including those which are characteristic of dyslexics. Among the founders were many social activists and others with nontraditional viewpoints. It will be remembered that the school was begun by parents, many of whom were children of founders of an arts and crafts community, and also by members of the Swarthmore College faculty community. As time went on, the school attracted similar families from the surrounding area. As a founding parent I had always valued these connections but was not fully aware of an extra dimension of insight it had given me in the course of this study.

Although it may be true, as the proverb goes, that the last person we should ask about the nature of water is the fish who takes it for granted, it is quite obvious that once that fish becomes aware of the medium of his existence, no one is in a better position to tell more about the make-up of his aquatic environment. Finally, as the question of incidence kept recurring, a film dropped from this fish's eyes and a missing part of the answer to the problem became clearer. Only after my 1990 insight into the importance of the uniqueness of the SRV constituency matrix did I fully realize the advantage of my intimate membership in the core community. By reason of having been so much a part of that matrix, I have known it in more detail than could any other possible student of this particular longitudinal data. At the same time, my training in teaching and my persistent vigilance against personal bias in judgment have, I believe, made it possible for me to look at the matrix and myself in it with a good degree of detachment and objectivity. This combination adds another unusual feature to the study's illumination of its area of research interest and somewhat allays the concern about the high level of incidence of dyslexia in the study's families. Richard L Masland, M.D., who has followed this analysis since its inception in 1963 with professional and personal interest, said upon reviewing the current text, "I think that you are very wise in this chapter to emphasize that the population from which these persons were selected is a very unusual one, easily accounting for the high incidence of dyslexia which you have observed."

SUMMARY

In this chapter we have turned our attention as far as possible especially to the aspects of the field of dyslexia which related to this study. For illustration I have used events and relationships in the lives of people with whom the reader has, by now, some sense of familiarity. At the same time I have indicated how the fresh light of new knowledge made clearer hitherto puzzling aspects of phenomena already observed, or marginally within my field of awareness.

Tracing changes to some of their roots and speculating on future possibilities are tempting activities for contemplation. Their foundation seems even firmer because of the conclusions drawn from the research-oriented fact finding and presentation of Part I and the more informally treated history and observations recounted in Part II. Whatever else we can glean, I think we can say with confidence that multisensory teaching within the framework of holistic education was successful, in this instance, and that the beneficial results have held up over time. This, I think, justifies a good measure of the optimism we may continue to feel in the field of dyslexia.

Chapter X

GENERALIZATIONS:
THE STUDY'S SIGNIFICANCE

IMPACT: WHAT WE HAVE SEEN AND HEARD

In this final summary, we look at the study's accomplishments and its implications for the future. Having justified its hypothesis in the scientific paradigm in Part I, the study has continued to chronicle the later years of its subjects' lives with narrative and descriptive detail to give further evidence of their eventual success and achievement, and of other biographical outcomes.

Reports of the study's impact on the climate of public opinion have come back by word-of-mouth, in print and in citations by other authors. Its story has reached, first of all, parents and clinicians to whom it was originally directed. To parents, and to dyslexics themselves, the study's message has brought relief and hope and has been a stimulus to action. The results have become increasingly known both to lay people and to professionals in the field of dyslexia and related disciplines. Clinical diagnosticians have been encouraged by its findings to give more optimistic prognoses. Educators in the field have been able to see in the account an example, sometimes a model, to use in developing their own programs. In Part I more conventionally formulated statements describing empirical data and their putative significance, the study has explicitly demonstrated connections between scientific research and related pragmatic procedures. During the past quarter-century, the study's results have become more widely known through the Orton Dyslexia Society and related educational and scientific organizations in the United States and other countries, notably in Canada, the United Kingdom, and the Czech Republic. What we have seen, heard, and experienced as a result of all this has reinforced my own opinion in line with what Orton said in 1946 (see page 63). I, likewise, believe we can say that whether or not the initial theory was correct or sufficient, it has led to educational principles and practices which alleviate or remediate the problems caused by what we now know as developmental dyslexia.

As the study's report draws to a conclusion, I believe we can say with increased assurance that, given proper identification, diagnosis, and education tailored to their special needs, dyslexic individuals can flourish throughout their lifetimes. At best, such a holistic education is one that combines developing competence in learning in general and in language-learning in particular; that fosters a sense of belonging in a community and values one's contribution to it; that transmits one's cultural heritage; and that inculcates an optimism for the future. The program I have described here was fortunate enough to be used in a school thoughtfully planned to meet the differing needs (academic, practical, social, and emotional) of all its children. The ways in which the program accomplished this for the children in this study, dyslexic and nondyslexic alike, have been shown in the preceding chapters of this book.

THE TEST OF TIME

It seems to me, and to many others in our field, that all students can develop language proficiency, especially in reading, commensurate with the levels of their innate intelligence. Motivation for growth is natural, but the will to learn may need to be rekindled if it has been compromised by circumstances beyond the learner's control, for in that case the outcomes may be incomplete or disappointing. The achievement of competence in language skills is a strong force for sustaining or reawakening the determination to succeed in accomplishing one's purposes at each developmental level. Reports on pragmatically utilized principles, with illustrative case histories, can be convincingly influential in improving language teaching services to persons in need of them, helping in ways that will not interfere with any student's broader education but will complement it. The prescription suggested by our study is not proposed as a panacea. However, even critics who were formerly skeptical now seem to look at the study's implications in a more favorable light. The value of the approach has been attested to by the lifetime of academic, professional, and occupational achievements of the participants in the study and their accompanying enthusiasm for living and enjoyment of the results of their efforts.

PRACTICAL APPLICATIONS

The impact of the study has been felt especially in the relationship between the field of dyslexia and trends in educational practice and opinion. The acceptability of the Orton approach and variations stemming from it have been more convincing because of the report's careful particularity of observation and the length of time it has covered. Further evidence of the impact of the study on the acceptability of its educational implications is to be seen, one way or another, in the curricula and practices of a variety of public and private schools. Of course, The School in Rose Valley experiment is by no means the only example from which other schools have drawn, but it was one of the very earliest whole-school models. Some other schools more recently established have been set up *primarily* for the education of dyslexic children and other students in need of intensive help with basic language development. Still other schools and clinics incorporate dyslexia services as one of their several special educational offerings.

As an example of the study's connection with the present-day educational scene, I have chosen to speak here in some detail of the Jemicy School, near Baltimore, Maryland, because, as of our 1990 data collection, it so closely resembles its self-chosen School in Rose Valley prototype. Convinced by my 1968 report, the parent founders and first educational directors of the Jemicy venture were influenced deliberately to use the experience of The School in Rose Valley to provide guidance for their new school. More than any other school with which I am familiar, Jemicy School has shaped its philosophy and curriculum after those of The School in Rose Valley as described in Part I, and thus given us an opportunity for pertinent comparisons.[1]

---

[1] This time factor should be kept in mind. Closely similar still in basic philosophy, each school has developed in its own way, with some differences of curricula and practices. The School in Rose Valley is still a privileged place in which to spend a happy and productive childhood and is a beneficial influence in the educational world. Comparison of the two schools as they are at present would be, however interesting and pleasant to contemplate, outside this volume's purpose.

From the founding of Jemicy School, its accepted *Philosophy* (see Appendix B) has been based on The School in Rose Valley experience, and to it Jemicy School has consciously and persistently subscribed in study and practice.

Jemicy School was, by 1990, eighteen years old, and there has been time to see parallel ways in which the two schools developed. It is notable that in institutional design both schools, although nearly forty years apart in their inception, were parent founded and professionally staffed. The author was a co-founder of both schools, in the former primarily as a parent and in the latter as a professional consultant and staff member. There were, and still are, some differences in the clientele of the two schools, but in both cases their location in the open suburbs of their respective metropolitan areas was chosen to serve their total educational purposes. At the beginning, in each case, a parent family generously lent its former home to provide buildings and grounds to house the new school. Frugal management of the meager tuition and contribution income under each school's first Board of Directors enabled its respective school to weather the early and very difficult stages. There has been strength over time in the responsible way in which each Board has provided fiscal management which has enabled the school head to concentrate on educational and administrative functions. In pedagogical matters, the problem of dyslexia *became a part of* The School in Rose Valley for the relevant individuals of its whole population, but dyslexia *was the central issue* in the minds of those who established Jemicy School. It is in several ways important to the story told here that the overall excellence of the schools' curricula was paramount in both cases.

At The School in Rose Valley research was developed *ex post facto*, while at Jemicy School formally designed research is in progress. For both populations there are carefully kept records of each student's academic and personal growth. Preliminary reports from Jemicy's present director indicate that its research, so far, reports outcomes consistent with those achieved by the entire School in Rose Valley cohort (which, the reader is reminded, had included students with the full range of language learning facility). These newer findings include variables associated with the language competence of Jemicy School graduates and their further educational achievements, occupational status, and feelings about quality of life. Such information supports the central thesis of this study: proper diagnosis, timely intervention, and appropriate instruction can obviate many of the problems associated with dyslexia. Dyslexia-related *problems* can be prevented, and *minds*, however constituted, from eulexic to dyslexic, can be significantly helped toward optimum functioning. However, *to speak of "preventing" or "curing" dyslexia itself would show continued misunderstanding of its fundamental constitutional nature.*

PEDAGOGY SUMMARIZED

My experience, begun at The School in Rose Valley, developed into a rationale for teaching that was adapted and shared throughout the widespread Orton-oriented community. The parameters of its empiric-theoretical approach, as described in Chapter 9, are compiled under four rubrics: the personal differences, the clinical diagnosis, the educational treatment, and the empathetic and scientific understanding of the problems of dyslexia.

Given this foundation, there seems naturally to follow the multidisciplinary approach to understanding and teaching which we have described as consistent with the designation of dyslexia as a field rather than as a single discipline. Using the knowledge and skill of experts in education, medicine, psychology, sociology, and linguistics, logic seems to require that the approach to the teaching of language be systematic, sequential and cumulative, and tailored to the cognitive and emotional needs of the individual student. What we say here is applicable to the teaching of a language that is, like English, characterized by an alphabetic-phonetic base. Like any other language, it needs to be learned by employing the human sensory modalities in an integrated, coordinated fashion. The aim is increasing mastery of language that can be employed for further learning and communication.

TEACHER EDUCATION

Of course, skilled teaching is vital to optimal results, and so a high order of teacher preparation is called for. At The School in Rose Valley, in training assistant tutors and teachers, who were mostly parent volunteers, in the Orton-Gillingham methodology, I used a consultative and apprenticeship approach. At that time, almost entirely unaware of Orton, teachers colleges did not train such instructors. (Since then there have been changes in a few universities, although teacher preparation is still far from ideal in our field.) On the basis of the Rose Valley experience, I was later able to develop an advanced level university course in the identification and teaching of language-learning disabled students of all ages. As my experience grew, I became increasingly convinced that a college level course including theory and practice would be more effective than the apprentice-type training I had previously utilized. My first such basic course was offered at Hood College in Frederick, Maryland, in 1959, and has been the foundation of further avenues of professional teacher preparation. Since that time numerous courses, my own and others, concerning the nature, identification, and treatment of dyslexia have been offered on a few college and university campuses elsewhere. Introductory lectures, workshops, and in-service sessions are now more readily available, and open to a broader range of teachers and others interested in the field.

EMPATHY AND UNDERSTANDING

In our informal four-fold taxonomy of dyslexia, "empathetic" is subsumed under "understanding," although it should actually be thought of as suffusing interpersonal relations in the whole domain. Semantically this is but another instance of the fact that it is not so much *life*, in the larger sense, as *our discourse about it* that lends itself to neatly segregated categories. My belief in the importance of empathy is reflected in the spirit of the foregoing chapters of this volume. The recognition and acceptance of commonality and difference among individuals in the community as a central value in its ethos can be fostered in the school to incorporate the empathy necessary for dealing successfully with dyslexia and its often associated problems. Under common sense control, empathy is not sentimentality but a high order art form that blends knowledge, skill, and imagination into a kind of poetry of therapy. It shows itself variously in pervasive intuitive talent for interpersonal relations, and in the disciplined skill of any of the helping professions. Empathy is an understanding and constructive force in dealing with dyslexic aspects of individual lives and with the complications which often ensue when the basic condition is not adequately addressed. As with any other of our gifts, awareness of the quality or its salience comes and goes, but in the total matrix of our lives it is always there to be used in the service of whatever vision and wisdom we have. Practiced within the limitations of human frailty, I believe empathy was a benign and central force in the childhood of our study's subjects.

SCIENTIFIC RESEARCH AND EDUCATIONAL TREATMENT

One of the strongest trends in the half-century during which this study has taken place has been the growth of scientific research. Both scientists and practitioners recognize that at the present stage there are significant gaps between basic biological knowledge and service given to individuals. Scientific research in the field of dyslexia has also pointed out the areas where we have long seen the need for further investigation. As practitioners we have learned much from the advances in the sciences while as scientists we have often recognized applications of scientific advances in the work done by practitioners. Some of us work at the same time as scientific researchers and educators. Time, space, and resources have limited discussion here of the extent and variety of both the increase in the understanding and the ongoing need. Although we sometimes fail to do so, both as scientists and as educators, I believe we should look for ways to encourage two-way traffic on the bridge between research findings and practice with people. Colleagues using similar approaches can find pertinent, often corroborative, evidence germane to their own work, evidence which has not always been apparent to them in their separate worlds. For example, it is often said in conclusions to scientific reports that their "findings will give us methods of treatment which will address the problems of dyslexia." Such researchers seem to be unaware of the connection between their work and treatments already in use. Successful clinical and educational practitioners need to find ways to communicate better with their research peers whose views usually are bounded within the theoretical and scientific arena. There is a need for cross-fertilization between the findings of neuroscientists and the applications of time-tested principles of educational practitioners. It is hard, if not impossible, to keep up with either field, let alone both! It has been my purpose and hope in some measure to contribute toward bridging the gaps we all see, share, and care about. For as Robert Frost in "Stopping by Woods on a Snowy Evening," put it, "[We] have promises to keep / And miles to go before [we] sleep."

CHANGE AND HOPE

As I end this study and look toward the future, I reflect particularly on changes seen and hopes engendered. Life is full of change, and as it zigzags its way forward, perhaps this account may serve as one example of the ways that an individual can open and further alert more people to those changes. The range of the study's time and subject matter is broad enough to speak to the interests of a wide variety of readers, including people in the whole of society on whose shoulders rests the responsibility for the educational transmission of its culture.

With all that is happening in the field of dyslexia, it is necessary in summarizing here to keep the focus on this study and its origins and effects. The earlier account has already helped to extend its message of justified optimism and hope in widening circles, through such avenues as: the study's own 1968 form; schools, somewhat in proportion with my personal involvement with them; the teaching of teachers, who, in turn, teach others; personal contacts of all sorts; the printed word; and now this new edition bringing my story into the present and particularly underscoring the robustness over time of the original results.

Dyslexia, however defined, has also reached the media, on the coattails of public interest in the handicapped and the atmosphere of social and educational crisis. We need continually to reinforce the idea that dyslexia is about the human mind and its constitution and that it is largely independent of categorical distinctions like ethnicity, social status, or personal characteristics; it cuts across them all. The "middle-class myth" we sometimes hear about is itself a myth. Dyslexia, undue lack of language facility, is as real, and potentially as devastating, to those whose life circumstances are in other respects propitious as it is to those we euphemistically call "disadvantaged." On the positive side, the productive and creative potentialities, the variability in language traits that are common among dyslexic persons and in dyslexia-prone families (our study's personnel noticeably included), are extended and intensified. They, also, one might say, are "category-blind." In terms of social ecology we impoverish both our students and ourselves unless we foster their giftedness at the same time that we are helping them overcome their ineptitudes. The term "gifted dyslexic" is far from being an oxymoron. This has been amply illustrated in history, in biographies of the famous, and is surely exemplified in our own small study's biographical excerpts.

When our subjects were children, we could already see in the general population that dozens and scores of people with dyslexia had been helped by appropriate diagnosis and remediation. Now, all over the country and in the wider world, we see hundreds, even thousands, of such instances, but this does not blind us to the millions who are still unserved or under-served. We are constantly reminded of them by frustrated children, distraught parents, and harassed educators, whose plight is so often the consequence of unresolved dyslexia problems. Many are the stories of a miserable childhood, emotional stress, and socioeconomic hardship or failure, and the persistence of lives of quiet or unquiet, often secretive, desperation. "Success against all odds" is also often heroic; its recognition and suitably publicized awards help to bind up wounds and to increase public awareness of needs, but even there we too often see emotional scar tissue. Examples such as this study show that the scar tissue and waste of potential can be forestalled. We can say "yes" and "speed the day" to more and better research, but "no" to delay of action until its results are in. *Today's children, with only one childhood granted to them, cannot wait for tomorrow's answers, nor do they need to do so!* Still with much to learn, we already know, and have known at least since our cohort's school days, enough to teach any child to speak, read, and write his own language, and we know how important it is to get more and more teachers ready to teach him and his schoolmates and their hitherto untaught elders. More research and improved methodology can bring us closer to the goals we see as within reach, but it is *now* that society needs exponential increase in educational effort.

DIAGNOSIS CONFIRMED; PROGNOSIS ASSURED

It is toward the liberation of the individual human capacities through which dreams and possibilities can be realized that our work has been directed. One can talk of possibilities in general terms, but it is individual persons, in all their variety, who dream the dreams, make the discoveries, revive old truths, and envision the new ones they may bring into being. It is the innate capacity in each person that society needs to nurture, as individuals discover their full selfhood through their own experience within each single human lifetime. In accordance with the Geschwind mandate, I have structured this report to present a scientific view of developmental dyslexia as seen through the eyes of one who has worked directly with dyslexic persons. This study, by its example, has tried to throw its ray of light on how such individual forces can be liberated and fostered. It presents one illustration of what *can be achieved* under reasonably informed and nurturing circumstances, by telling its own story of what *has actually been achieved* in the real world.

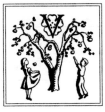

THE SCHOOL IN ROSE VALLEY

School Lane, Moylan. PA 19065 • (215) 566-1088

60th Anniversary

Name: _____

Address: _____

Date of Birth: _____ Sex: _____

Father's Name: _____ Occupation: _____

Mother's Name: _____ Occupation: _____

Marital Status: _____ Spouse's Name: _____

Children? (Names & Ages): _____

_____

_____

_____

Other family members who attended SRV: _____

_____

_____

What other schools did you attend?

Elementary: _____

Jr. High: _____

High School: _____

College: _____

Graduate or Professional School: _____

Highest Degree Earned: _____

Present Employment: _____

Past Employment: _____

_____

_____

Civic Activities/Interests/Hobbies: _____

_____

_____

_____

ROSE VALLEY EDUCATION:

What grades did you attain at SRV? _____

What was your last year at SRV (ex. 1980)? _____

Memorable Teachers: _____

_____

_____

_____

Memorable Activities: _____

_____

_____

_____

How did transition to later schooling go? What was hard? What was easy? _____

_____

_____

_____

_____

How did SRV influence later life experiences? _____

_____

_____

_____

_____

Have you kept in touch with SRV or your classmates? _____

_____

_____

_____

Signature: _____   Date: _____

SRV 1989 QUESTIONNAIRE

(Significant happenings in your life since, let's say, 1960.)

Name _____

Address _____

Phone _____

Advanced Study

    Where & how many years _____

    Degrees—dates & sources _____

Present occupation & job title _____

    High points in career _____

    Significant career changes & when _____

Special honors, any kind _____

Publications, inventions, etc. _____

Martial status _____

    Name of spouse _____

Descendants—names, birth-years, schooling, occupations, families, etc.

_____

_____

_____

_____

Comment on any holdover school-related problems _____

_____

_____

    Any among your descendants? _____

    _____

    _____

    _____

Avocational interests: do you enjoy

Reading? _____

Speaking? _____

Writing? _____

Dealing with figures? _____

Making things? _____

Other Delights or bug-aboos? _____

Which of your achievements give you most satisfaction? _____

_____

_____

Do you have a recent snapshot or so to share?

Did you get to read the 1968 study about all of you (*Developmental Dyslexia: Adult Achievements of Dyslexic* (and Nondyslexic) *Boys*)? _____

What else should I have asked you? _____

_____

_____

_____

Thank You!
Margaret

APPENDIX B

THE SCHOOL AT JEMICY FARM

A Philosophy

A school should be designed for its children, their present happy growth and their soundly based future effectiveness. A school is established as a *group* in which people are taught or led to learn, but it is as *individuals* that they learn, through experiencing group life and developing unique personal competences and understanding of their world.

Just as, in Aldous Huxley's words, "It is no good knowing about the taste of strawberries out of a book," so each child needs to experience for himself the worlds of city and country, of nature and human culture. These become part of him through all his senses, through emotional and spiritual appreciation and responsible involvement in all the world about and within him, and by the active processes of the ordered observation, problem solving, and critical thinking which we call intellectual functioning.

Each child is born with a distinctive combination of potentialities on which, by the time he comes to school, a unique set of experiences has been at work making him a separate individual, different from all others. At the same time, he is a member of the human family, with certain basic physical, emotional, and spiritual characteristics and needs which he shares with all of us. It is this which makes society both necessary and possible. A school life which promotes the healthy, vigorous, joyful growth of its children should provide a well-planned physical setting and general program. Such dependable security gives a firm foundation and a stable framework within which each child can live a cooperative and rewarding social life while he is developing from dependent childhood into self-reliant adolescence and adulthood.

But this provides only the background for the major interest of the school, which is the meeting of each child's specific needs and the fostering of his strengths and unique talents. The plan which is best for him is the one which will enable him to grow toward achieving his own potentialities. For this he needs a richly varied educational experience in physical activity and sports, in a wide variety of creative arts, in happy social relationships, and in the intellectual appreciation of his cultural heritage.

He needs careful training, too, in the basic skills which are the tools through whose use he will develop competence and a sense of confidence in achieving his educational objectives. Tools themselves are not the goals of education, but just as it is difficult or impossible to construct a beautiful and satisfying building without a set of well-sharpened tools and the skill to use them, so one cannot hope to acquire knowledge, understanding, and vocational competence without mastery of reading, writing, mathematics, and the disciplines imposed by shop, studio, laboratory, and playing field.

Children have varied degrees of talent and difficulty in different traits, and so their needs differ. Wholeness of development requires that we know a child's strengths so that we may encourage him to use them well, and know, too, the exact nature of his difficulties so that we may help him to cope successfully with them, and so gain a well-rounded competence as an effective person.

To achieve these goals for the school there must be a staff which itself embodies wholeness of body, mind, and spirit, with a capacity for both loving acceptance and calm firmness. Effective pedagogy requires knowledge and enthusiasm in subject matter, coupled with astute assessment of individual children's needs and capacities and skill in teaching each one in his own style and at his own pace, whether individually or in varying groups.

Since none of us is all-knowing, the planning and operation of the school requires not only teamwork on the campus but also consultation with outside experts when needed, cooperation of parents, and, most important, a spirit of involvement on the part of the children as they grow toward taking full responsibility for their own behavior and learning.

This is education—a leading forth—toward the full, happy, and effective living we all want for each of our children and for the school community as a whole. This experience of the good life in childhood, with the development of competence and adaptability, is the best preparation we know for meeting the demands of later schooling and of a world of rapid change and complexity. Specific training is obsolete before it is mastered, but intellectual curiosity, skill in learning, and creative flexibility in the face of new problems are dependable resources with which to meet whatever the future may hold of challenge and opportunity.

These are the objectives to which *the School at Jemicy Farm* has dedicated itself.

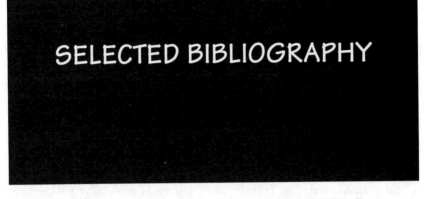

SELECTED BIBLIOGRAPHY

Akin, F. 1913. *Word Mastery*. New York: Houghton, Mifflin Co.

Annals of Dyslexia: An Interdisciplinary Journal of The Orton Dyslexia Society. 1989. Volume XXXIX. Baltimore: The Orton Dyslexia Society. (This volume contains several papers whose contents and authors seem particularly relevant to the readers of my 1995 edition.)

Annett, M. 1985. *Left, Right, Hand and Brain: The Right Shift Theory*. Hillsdale, NJ: Lawrence Erlbaum Associates.

Ansara, A., N. Geschwind, A. Galaburda, M. Albert, and N. Gartrell, eds. 1981. *Sex Differences in Dyslexia*. Towson, MD: The Orton Dyslexia Society.

Arthur, G. 1946. *Tutoring as Therapy*. New York: Commonwealth Fund.

Bakker, D. J. 1990. *Neuropsychological Treatment of Dyslexia*. New York: Oxford University Press.

Balmuth, M. 1982. *The Roots of Phonics: A Historical Introduction*. Baltimore: McGraw-Hill.

Balow, B. and M. Blomquist. 1965. "Young adults ten to fifteen years after severe reading disability." *Elementary School Journal*. 66: 44–48.

Barzun, J. 1959. *The House of Intellect*. New York: Harper & Bros.

Barzun, J. and H. F. Graff. 1957. *The Modern Researcher*. New York: Harcourt, Brace & Co.

Berlyne, D. E. 1966. "Conflict and arousal." *Scientific American*, 215: 82–87.

Berstein, J. 1963. *The Analytic Engine: Computers-Past, Present and Future*. New York: Random House.

Betts, E. A. 1936. *The Prevention and Correction of Reading Difficulties*. Evanston, IL: Row, Peterson and Co.

Brady, S. A. and D. P. Shankweiler. 1991. *Phonological Processes in Lit-*

eracy: A Tribute to Isabelle Y. Liberman. Hillsdale, NJ: Lawrence Erlbaum Associates.

Bronner, A. F. 1917. *The Psychology of Special Abilities and Disabilities.* Boston: Little, Brown.

Brown, R. 1958. *Words and Things.* Glencoe, IL: Free Press.

Bruner, J. 1961. *The Process of Education.* Cambridge, MA: Harvard University Press.

Cole, E. M. and L. Walker. 1964. "Reading and speech problems as expressions of a specific language disability." *Disorders of Communications,* Vol. XLII; Research Publications, A.R.N.M.D. New York: Association for Research in Nervous and Mental Disease.

Cremin, L. A. 1961. *The Transformation of the School.* New York: Alfred A. Knopf.

Critchley, M. 1964. *Developmental Dyslexia.* Springfield, IL: Charles C. Thomas.

———. 1970. *The Dyslexic Child.* Springfield, IL: Charles C. Thomas.

———. 1975. *Silent Language.* London: Butterworths.

Critchley, M. and E. Critchley. 1978. *Dyslexia Defined.* Springfield, IL: Charles C. Thomas.

de Hirsch, K., J. J. Jansky, and W. S. Langford. 1966. *Predicting Reading Failure.* New York: Harper and Row.

Demarest, A. J. and W. Van Sickle. 1900. *New Education Readers: A Synthetic and Phonic Word Method.* New York: American Book Company.

Dewey, J. 1913. *Interest and Effort in Education.* New York: Houghton, Mifflin.

Drew, A. L. 1956. "A neurological appraisal of familial congenital word-blindness." *Brain,* 79: 440–460.

Duane, D. D. and M. B. Rawson, eds. 1974. *Reading, Perception and Language: Papers from the World Congress on Dyslexia.* Baltimore: York Press.

Duffy, F., M.D. and Geschwind, N., M.D., eds. 1985. *Dyslexia: A Neuroscientific Approach to Clinical Evaluation.* Boston: Little, Brown and Company.

Edelman, G. M. 1992. *Bright Air, Brilliant Fire: On the Matter of the Mind.* New York: Basic Books.

Eisenberg, L. 1966. "The epidemiology of reading retardation and a program for preventive intervention." In *The Disabled Reader: Education of the Dyslexic Child,* edited by J. Money, Baltimore: The Johns Hopkins Press.

Ellis, W., ed. 1991. *All Language and the Creation of Literacy.* Baltimore: The Orton Dyslexia Society, Inc.

———. 1988. *Intimacy with Language: A Forgotten Basic in Teacher Education.* Baltimore: The Orton Dyslexia Society.

Erikson, E. H. 1959. "Identity and the life cycle." *Psychological Issues,* Vol. 1, No. 1, Monograph No. 1. New York: International Universities Press, Inc.

Fernald, G. M. 1988. *Remedial Techniques in Basic School Subjects.* Austin: Pro-ed.

Finucci, J. M., L. S. Gottsfredson, and B. Childs. 1986. "A follow-up study of dyslexic boys." *Annals of Dyslexia: An Interdisciplinary Journal of The Orton Dyslexia Society.* Volume XXXV. Baltimore: The Orton Dyslexia Society.

Flower, R. M., H. F. Gofman, and L. I. Lawson, eds. 1965. *Reading Disorders: A Multidisiplinary Symposium.* Philadelphia: F. A. Davis Co.

Galaburda, A. M. 1989. "Ordinary and Extraordinary Brain Development: Anatomical Variation in Developmental Dyslexia." *Annals of Dyslexia: An Interdisciplinary Journal of The Orton Dyslexia Society.* Volume XXXIX. Baltimore: The Orton Dyslexia Society.

Galaburda, A. M., ed. 1993. *Dyslexia and Development: Neurobiological Aspects of Extra-Ordinary Brains.* Cambridge, MA: Harvard University Press.

———. 1989. *From Reading to Neurons.* Cambridge, MA: The MIT Press.

Galaburda, A. and N. Geschwind, eds. 1985. *Cerebral Lateralization: Biological Mechanisms, Associations, and Pathology.* Cambridge, MA: The MIT Press.

Gallagher, J. R. 1948. "Can't read can't spell." *The Atlantic Monthly,* 181: 35–39.

———. 1960. "Specific language disability (dyslexia)." *Clin. Proc. of the Children's Hosp.,* 16: 1, 3–15.

Gardner, H. 1983. *Frames of Mind: The Theory of Multiple Intelligences.* New York: Basic Books, Inc.

Gates, A. I. 1949. *The Improvement of Reading.* New York: Macmillan (The 1935 edition was used by the author of this study in 1935–1947.)

Gillingham, A. and B. Stillman. 1936. *Remedial Training for Children with Specific Disability in Reading, Spelling and Penmanship.* New York: Privately published by the authors. (Two other editions, that of 1956 with red cover and that of 1960 with green cover, are now published by Educators Publishing Service, Inc. Cambridge, MA. The author used the 1936 edition at The School in Rose Valley.)

Ginsberg, E. and J. L. Herma and Associates. 1964. *Talent and Performance*. New York: Columbia University Press.

Goldstein, H. K. 1963. *Research Standards and Methods for Social Workers*. New Orleans: The Hauser Press.

Goldstein, K. 1939. *The Organism: A Holistic Approach to Biology Derived from Pathological Data in Man*. New York: American Book Co. (Paperback edition, 1963, Boston: Beacon.)

Gordon, M. M. 1950. *Social Class in American Sociology*. Durham, NC: Duke University Press. (Paperback edition, 1963, New York: McGraw-Hill.)

Gray, D. B. and J. F. Kavanagh, eds. 1983. *Biobehavioral Measures of Dyslexia*. Parkton, MD: York Press, Inc.

Gray, W. S. Undated. *Oral Reading Paragraphs* (test), Old Form. Bloomington, IL: Public School Publishing Co.

Guilford, J. P. 1965. *Fundamental Statistics in Psychology and Education*, 4th ed. New York: McGraw-Hill.

Haggerty, M.E. and M. E. Noonan. 1929. *Haggerty Reading Examination, Sigma 1*. New York: World Book Co.

Hall, E. T. 1959. *The Silent Language*. Garden City, NY: Doubleday.

Hallgren, B. 1950. "Specific dyslexia (congenital word-blindness)." *Acta Psychiat. Neurol. Scand. Suppl.*, 65: 1–287.

Head, H. 1926. *Aphasia and Kindred Disorders of Speech*. New York: Macmillan.

Hermann, K. 1959. *Reading Disability: A Medical Study of Word-Blindness and Related Handicaps*. trans. P. G. Aungle. Springfield, IL: Charles C. Thomas.

Henry, M. K. 1988. "Beyond Phonics: Integrated Decoding and Spelling Instruction Based on Word Origin and Structure." *Annals of Dyslexia: An Interdisciplinary Journal of The Orton Dyslexia Society*, Volume XXXVIII. Baltimore: The Orton Dyslexia Society.

————. 1964. "Specific reading disability, with special reference to complicated word blindness." *Danish Medical Bulletin*, 11: 34–40.

Hinshelwood, J. 1896. "A Case of dyslexia: a peculiar form of word-blindness." *Lancet* 2: 1451–4.

————. 1917. *Congenital Word Blindness*. London: H. K. Lewis.

Hollingworth, L. S. 1918. *The Psychology of Special Disability in Spell-*

ing. Contributions to Education No. 88. New York: Teachers College, Columbia University Press.

———. 1925. *Special Talents and Defects.* New York: Macmillan.

Johnson, W. 1946. *People in Quandaries.* New York: Harper.

Kavanagh, J. F. ed. 1991. *The Language Continuum: From Infancy to Literacy.* Parkton, MD: York Press, Inc.

Kerr, J. 1897. "School Hygiene in its mental, moral, and physical aspects." *J. Roy. Stat. Soc.* 60: 613–80.

Klasen, E. 1972. *The Syndrome of Specific Dyslexia: With Special Consideration of its Physiological, Psychological, Testpsychological, and Social Correlates.* Baltimore: University Park Press.

Kline, C. L. 1977. "Follow-up study of 216 dyslexic children." *Bulletin of The Orton Society, 25,* 127–144.

Lecky, P. 1945. *Self-Consistency.* New York: Island Press.

Liberman, A. M. 1989. "Reading is Hard Just Because Listening is Easy." In *Wenner-Gren International Symposium Series: Brain and Reading,* edited by C. von Euler, M.D. Hampshire, England: Macmillan.

Liberman, I. Y. 1988. "Language and Literacy: The Obligation of the Schools of Education." In *Intimacy with Language,* edited by W. Ellis. Baltimore: The Orton Dyslexia Society.

Livingstone, M. 1993. "Parallel Processing in the Visual System and the Brain: Is One Subsystem Selectively Affected in Dyslexia?" In *Dyslexia and Development: Neurobiological Aspects of Extra-Ordinary Brains,* edited by A. M. Galaburda. Cambridge, MA: Harvard University Press.

Masland, R. L. and M. W. Masland, eds. 1988. *Preschool Prevention of Reading Failure.* Parkton, MD: York Press.

Masland, R. L. 1967. "Brain mechanisms underlying the language function." *Bulletin of the Orton Society,* 17: 1–31.

Matejcek, Z. 1994. *Dyslexie: Specificke Poruchy Cteni.* Prague: H&H.

McClelland, J. 1989. "Gillingham: Contemporary after 76 Years." *Annals of Dyslexia: An Interdisciplinary Journal of The Orton Dyslexia Society.* Volume XXXIX. Baltimore: The Orton Dyslexia Society.

McCormick, E.M. 1958. *Digital Computer Primer.* New York: McGraw-Hill.

Money, J., ed. 1962. *Reading Disability: Progress and Research Needs in Dyslexia.* Baltimore: The Johns Hopkins Press.

———. 1966. *The Disabled Reader: Education of the Dyslexic Child.* Baltimore: The Johns Hopkins Press.

Monroe, M. 1932. *Children Who Cannot Read.* Chicago: University of Chicago Press.

Monroe, M. and B. Backus. 1937. *Remedial Reading.* New York: Houghton, Mifflin.

Morgan W. P. 1896. "A case of congenital word-blindness." *Brit. Med. J.* 2: 1378.

Njiokiktjien, C. 1993. "Neurological Arguments for a Joint Developmental Dysphasia-Dyslexia Syndrome." In *Dyslexia and Development: Neurological Aspects of Extra-Ordinary Brains,* edited by A. M. Galaburda. Cambridge, MA: Harvard University Press.

Nowell, F., Jr. 1966. Grace Rotzel, *Parents' Bulletin of The School in Rose Valley,* 274: 4.

Orton, J. L. 1964. *A Guide to Teaching Phonics.* Cambridge, MA: Educators Publishing Service, Inc.

———. 1966a. "The Orton-Gillingham Approach." In *The Disabled Reader: Education of the Dyslexic Child,* edited by J. Money. Baltimore: The Johns Hopkins Press.

———, ed. 1966b. *"Word-Blindness" in School Children and Other Papers on Strephosymbolia (Specific Language Disability – Dyslexia) 1925–1946.* Monograph No. 2 of The Orton Society. Pomfret, CT: The Orton Society.

Orton, S. T. 1925. "Word-blindness in school children." *Archives of Neurology and Psychiatry,* 14: 581–615.

———. 1928. "Specific reading disability-strephosymbolia." *Journal American Medical Assn.,* 90:14, 1095–1099. (Reprinted, 1928, *Bulletin of the Orton Society,* 13: 9–17; also reprinted in Orton, J. L. 1966b.)

———. 1937. *Reading, Writing and Speech Problems in Children.* New York: W. W. Norton.

———. 1989. *Reading, Writing, and Speech Problems in Children and Selected Papers.* Austin: Pro-Ed.

Partridge, E. 1959. *Origins.* New York: Macmillan

Pavlidis, G. T. and T. R. Miles, eds. 1981. *Dyslexia Research and its Applications to Education.* New York: John Wiley & Sons.

Pavlidis, G. T. and D. F. Fisher, eds. 1986. *Dyslexia: Its Neuropsychology and Treatment.* New York: John Wiley & Sons.

Peatman, J. G. 1947. *Descriptive and Sampling Statistics.* New York: Harper.

Penfield, W. and L. Roberts. 1959. *Speech and Brain Mechanisms.* Princeton, NJ: Princeton University Press.

Preston, R. C. and D. J. Yarington. 1966. "Status of fifty retarded readers eight years after reading clinic diagnosis." University of Pennsylvania. Unpublished paper.

Rabinovitch, R. D. 1962. "Dyslexia: psychiatric considerations." In *Reading Disability: Progress and Research Needs in Dyslexia,* edited by J. Money. Baltimore: The Johns Hopkins Press.

Rawson, M. B. 1966a. "Prognosis in dyslexia." *Academic Therapy Quarterly* 1: 164–173.

———. 1966b. "After a generation's time: a follow-up study of fifty-six boys: a preliminary report." *Bulletin of The Orton Society,* 16: 24–37.

———. 1966c. *A Bibliography on the Nature, Recognition and Treatment of Language Difficulties.* Pomfret, CT: The Orton Society.

———. 1968. *Developmental Language Disability: Adult Accomplishments of Dyslexic Boys.* 1st ed. Baltimore: The Johns Hopkins Press.

———. 1978. *Developmental Language Disability: Adult Accomplishments of Dyslexic Boys.* 2nd ed. Cambridge, MA: Educators Publishing Service, Inc.

———. 1974. *A Bibliography on the Nature, Recognition and Treatment of Language Difficulties.* Baltimore: The Orton Society, Inc.

———. 1988. *The Many Faces of Dyslexia.* Baltimore: The Orton Dyslexia Society.

Richardson, R. B. and M. Monsour, eds. 1979. *Dilemmas of Dyslexia.* Charlottesville, NC: The Charlottesville Center for Dyslexia.

Richardson, S. O. 1991. "The Alphabetic Principle: Roots of Literacy." In *All Language and the Creation of Literacy,* edited by W. Ellis. Baltimore: The Orton Dyslexia.

Robinson, H. M. and H. K. Smith. 1962. "Reading clinic clients—ten years after." *Elementary School Journal,* 63: 22–27.

Roe, A. 1952. *The Making of a Scientist.* New York: Dodd, Mead.

Rosenthal, R. and L. Jacobson. 1968. *Pygmalion in the Classroom: Teacher Expectation and Pupils' Intellectual Development.* New York: Holt, Rinehart and Winston, Inc.

Rotzel, G. 1971. *The School in Rose Valley: A Parent Venture in Education.* Baltimore: The Johns Hopkins Press.

Saunders, R. E. 1962. "Dyslexia: its phenomenology." In *Reading Disability: Progress and Research Needs in Dyslexia,* edited by J. Money. Baltimore: The Johns Hopkins Press.

Sherrington, C. 1940. *Man on His Nature.* Cambridge, England: Cambridge University Press.

Silver, A. A. and R. A. Hagin. 1964. "Specific reading disability: follow-up studies." *Am. Jour. Orthopsychiatry,* 34: 95–102.

———. 1990. *Disorders of Learning in Childhood.* New York: John Wiley & Sons.

Smelt, E. D. 1976. *Speak, Spell and Read English.* Longmans Australia Pty. Ltd.

Sperry, R. W. 1964. "The great cerebral commissure." *Scientific American.* 210: 42–52.

Stanger, M. and E. Donohue. 1937. *Prediction and Prevention of Reading Difficulties.* New York: Oxford University Press.

Terman, L. M. and M. A. Merrill. 1937. *Measuring Intelligence.* New York: Houghton, Mifflin.

Terman, L. M. and M. H. Oden and Associates. 1947. *Genetic Studies of Genius, Vol IV, The Gifted Child Grows Up.* Stanford, CA: Stanford University Press.

———. 1959. *Genetic Studies of Genius, Vol. V. The Gifted Group at Mid-Life.* Stanford, CA: Stanford University Press.

Thompson, L. J. 1966. *Reading Disability: Developmental Dyslexia.* Springfield, IL: Charles C. Thomas.

Walker, L. and E. M. Cole. 1965. "Familial patterns of specific reading disability in a population sample: Part I-prevalence, distribution and persistence." *Bulletin of the Orton Society,* 15: 12–24.

Warner, W. L. with M. Meeker and K. Eels. 1949. *Social Class in America.* New York: Harper. (Paperback edition, 1960, New York: Harper Torchbooks.)

Wechsler, D. 1939. *Wechsler-Bellevue Intelligence Scale,* Form I. New York: Psychological Corporation.

———. 1949. *Wechsler Intelligence Scale for Children.* New York: Psychological Corporation.

West, T. G. 1991. *In the Mind's Eye: Visual Thinkers, Gifted People with Learning Difficulties, Computer Images, and the Ironies of Creativity.* Buffalo: Prometheus Books.

Zangwill, O. L. 1960. *Cerebral Dominance and Its Relation to Psychological Function.* London: Oliver & Boyd.

Zelditch, M., Jr. 1959. *A Basic Course in Sociological Statistics.* New York: Henry Holt.

Zerbin-Rudin, Edith. 1967. Kongenitale Wortblindheit oder Spezifische Dyslexie (Congenital word-blindness). In *Homangenetick,* Vol. V/2. Stuttgart, Germany: Thieme. Translation by Steven G. Vandenberg in *Bulletin of the Orton Society,* 17: 47–54 (1967).

INDEX TO PART ONE *

*Index to Part II has been postponed.